D0221871

*Procedures and
Documentation for
Mammography and
Quality Management*

NOTICE

Medicine is an ever-changing science. As new research and clinical experience broaden our knowledge, changes in treatment and drug therapy are required. The authors and the publisher of this work have checked with sources believed to be reliable in their efforts to provide information that is complete and generally in accord with the standards accepted at the time of publication. However, in view of the possibility of human error or changes in medical sciences, neither the authors not the publisher nor any other party who has been involved in the preparation or publication of this work warrants that the information contained herein is in every respect accurate or complete, and they are not responsible for any errors or omissions or for the results obtained from use of such information. Readers are encouraged to confirm the information contained herein with other sources. For example and in particular, readers are advised to check the product information sheet included in the package of each drug they plan to administer to be certain that the information contained in this book is accurate and that changes have not been made in the recommended dose or in the contraindications for administration. This recommendation is of particular importance in connection with new or infrequently used drugs.

Procedures and Documentation for Mammography and Quality Management

Series Editor:
Erica Koch Williams, M.Ed., R.T.(R)(M)(QM)
Assistant Professor of Allied Health,
Fort Hays State University, Hays, Kansas

Editor:
Jennifer Wagner, B.S., R.T.(R)(M)(QM)
Instructor of Allied Health,
Fort Hays State University, Hays, Kansas

McGRAW-HILL
HEALTH PROFESSIONS DIVISION

New York St. Louis San Francisco Auckland Bogotá Caracas Lisbon London Madrid Mexico City
Milan Montreal New Delhi San Juan Singapore Sydney Tokyo Toronto

McGraw-Hill

A Division of The McGraw·Hill Companies

**PROCEDURES AND DOCUMENTATION FOR
MAMMOGRAPHY AND QUALITY MANAGEMENT**

Copyright © 2000 by The **McGraw-Hill Companies,** Inc. All rights
reserved. Printed in the United States of America. Except as permitted
under the United States Copyright Act of 1976, no part of this
publication may be reproduced or distributed in any form or by any
means, or stored in a data base or retrieval system, without the prior
written permission of the publisher.

1 2 3 4 5 6 7 8 9 0 MAL MAL 99

ISBN 0-07-135398-4

This book was set in Times Roman and Optima by V&M Graphics, Inc.
The editors were John Dolan and Nicky Panton.
The production supervisor was Richard C. Ruzycka.
Malloy Lithographing, Inc. was printer and binder.

This book is printed on acid-free paper.

Cataloging-in-publication data is on file for this book at the Library of Congress.

Contents

Preface   *ix*
Acknowledgments   *xi*

PART ONE
Mammography

Chapter 1   Patient Education Proficiency Criteria   3

1. Compression   3
2. Personal History   4
3. Breast Self Examination (BSE)   5
4. Health Guidelines   7

Chapter 2   Technical Proficiency Criteria   9

1. Proper Technical Factors   9
2. Basic Tissue Types   10
3. Essential Imaging Evaluation   11

Chapter 3   Position Proficiency Criteria   15

1. Standard Views   15
2. Additional Projections   20
3. Modified Studies   31
4. Mammography of the Male Patient   39
5. Special Procedures   41

Chapter 4   Quality Control and Management Proficiency Criteria   **53**

1. Compression   53
2. Darkroom Cleanliness   55
3. Darkroom Fog   56
4. Film–Screen Contact   58
5. Fixer Retention   60
6. Phantom Imaging   62
7. Processor Quality Control   67
8. Repeat Analysis   71
9. Screen Cleanliness   73
10. View Box Uniformity   75
11. Visual Checklist   77

PART TWO
Quality Management

Introduction   **80**

Chapter 5   Equipment Evaluation   **83**

1. Automatic Exposure Control   83
2. Timer Evaluation   89
3. Half–Value Layer   93
4. Grid Uniformity Evaluation   95
5. Field Light Accuracy   96
6. Milliampere Linearity Evaluation   99
7. Milliamperage and Seconds Reciprocity   100
8. Milliampere Reproducibility   102
9. Kilovoltage Accuracy Evaluation   103
10. View Box Uniformity Evaluation   106

Chapter 6 **Mammography Quality Control Procedures** **109**

    1. Compression 109
    2. Darkroom Cleanliness 111
    3. Darkroom Fog 112
    4. Film–Screen Contact 114
    5. Fixer Retention 116
    6. Phantom Imaging 118
    7. Mammography Processor Quality Control 122
    8. Repeat Analysis 125
    9. Screen Cleanliness 127
    10. View–Box Uniformity 128
    11. Visual Checklist 130

Chapter 7 **Artifact Assessment** **131**

    1. Assessment 131
       a. Delay Streaks 132
       b. Entrance Roller Marks 132
       c. Guide Shoe Marks 132
       d. Chatter 133
       e. Dichroic Stain 133
       f. Brown Films 134
       g. Emulsion Pick–Off 134
       h. Skivings 134
       i. Curtain Effect 135
       j. Hyporetention 135
    2. Exposure Artifacts 135
       a. Motion 135
       b. Artifacts 135
       c. Poor Film-Screen Contact 136
       d. Grid Cut–Off 136
       e. Grid Lines 136
       f. Moiré Effect 136
       g. Quantum Mottle 136
    3. Storage and Handling Artifacts 136
       a. Age Fog 136
       b. Safelight Fog 136
       c. Pressure Marks 137
       d. Static 137
       e. Crescent or Crinkle Marks 137
       f. Shadow Images 137

Chapter 8 **Processor Quality Control**   **139**

1. Processor Quality Control   139
2. Components of Processing   141
3. Charting Processor QC   145
4. H & D Curves   148
5. Interpreting the Characteristic Curve   149
6. Silver Recovery   150
7. Materials Safety Data Sheet (MSDS)   151

Chapter 9 **Statistical Analysis**   **153**

1. Methods of Analyzing Data   153
2. Mathematical Description   154
   a. *Frequency*   154
   b. *Central Tendency*   154
3. Tools for Problem Identification and Analysis   155
4. Decision–Making Tools for Groups   159
5. Data Collection Methods and Indicators   162

Chapter 10 **Federal Regulations**   **165**

1. National Council on Radiation Protection and Measurements
   a. *Report Number 99: Quality Assurance for Diagnostic Imaging Equipment   165*
   b. *Report Number 105: Radiation Protection for Medical and Allied Health Personnel   166*

Appendices   **167**

1. Quick Reference to Test Frequency for Radiography   167
2. Quick Reference to Test Frequency for Mammography   168

Preface

This book is the first in a new McGraw-Hill series, which evolved to address the focus on competency and documentation in the advanced imaging modalities.

The text intends to be a supplement to the clinical components of Mammography and Quality Management. The authors realize that the methods of completing certain procedures are sometimes as diverse as the patients they serve. We have tried to formulate a step-by-step plan for each of the basic processes used by imaging professionals to achieve quality images in mammography. The Quality Management section includes both theory and analysis of common Quality Control tests and Quality Management philosophy. The design of the book should allow the professional, student and instructor greater ease in achieving and documenting competence in these fields of specialty. The appendix includes information on test frequency for diagnostic radiography and mammography. A separate section contains documentation forms to verify procedures accomplished.

We strongly encourage the user to apply their knowledge to complete all requirements in order to obtain advanced qualifications in their specialized modality. While advanced qualifications may not guarantee quality, they add credibility to the overall knowledge of the imaging professional. Competence can only be achieved through active participation, repetition and real interest in perfecting that which one does.

Erica Koch Williams
Jennifer Wagner

Acknowledgments

I wish to thank my colleagues, especially Jennifer Wagner, at Fort Hays State University for their input and encouragement on this work. This book is dedicated to my UMC companions from years gone by—Deshay Addison, Dirk Buys, Howard Epstein, Martin Gallacher, Chris Kennedy, and Katie Parker. You taught me through example what a competent imaging professional should be.

Erica Koch Williams

I would like to thank all the educators and trained professionals in the field who have helped instill the knowledge to get me where I am today. I would also like to thank my family, especially my husband Eric, for their support and encouragement through all my years of education and in my professional career.

Jennifer Wagner

Procedures and Documentation for Mammography and Quality Management

PART 1

Mammography

Chapter 1   Patient Education Proficiency Criteria
- Compression
- Personal History
- Breast Self-Examination
- Health Guidelines

Chapter 2   Technical Proficiency Criteria
- Proper Technical Factors
- Basic Tissue Types
- Essential Imaging Evaluation

Chapter 3   Position Proficiency Criteria

Standard Views
- Basic Principles
- Craniocaudal
- Mediolateral Oblique

Additional Projections
- Axillary Tail
- Cleavage View
- Exaggerated Craniocaudal
- 90° Mediolateral Projection
- 90° Lateromedial Projection
- Magnification Views
- Spot Images
- Tangential Projection

Modified Studies
- Augmented Breast
- Immobile Patient Positioning
- Positioning of the Large Breast
- Positioning of the Small Breast
- Postmastectomy Positioning

Mammography of the Male Patient
- Caudocranial Projection
- Mediolateral Oblique Projection

Special Procedures
- Needle Localization
- Ductography
- Fine-Needle Aspiration
- Magnetic Resonance Imaging
- Ultrasound
- Steriotactic Breast Biopsy

Chapter 4   *Quality Control and Management*
Proficiency Criteria
- Compression
- Darkroom Cleanliness
- Darkroom Fog
- Film–Screen Contact
- Fixer Retention
- Phantom Imaging
- Processor Quality Control
- Repeat Analysis
- Screen Cleanliness
- View Box Uniformity
- Visual Checklist

CHAPTER 1

Patient Education Proficiency Criteria

COMPRESSION

Compression devices should be constructed so that the posterior edges and the surface are straight, not rounded. The compression device should remain parallel to the image receptor at all times.

FIGURE 1-1

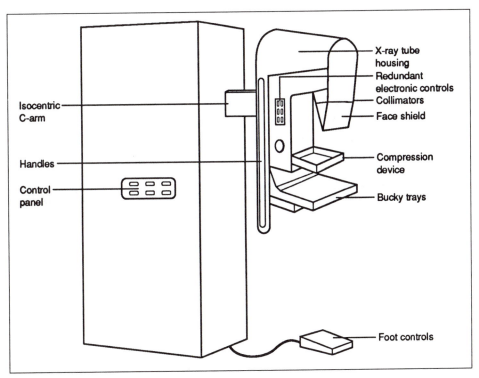

Terms

The American College of Radiology (ACR) defines *proper compression* as the maximum degree a patient's breast can be compressed and the amount of compression the patient can tolerate.

Minimal compression is the amount of compression required to bring the skin taunt. *Maximum compression* is the point at which compression becomes painful for the individual patient.

Reasons for Compression

- Reduces object image distance (OID)
- Allows for more uniform densities
- Reduces patient dose
- Separates breast structures
- Improves overall image sharpness

Proper Compression

Proper compression is achieved through exceptional patient care and a skilled imaging professional. Methods to achieve proper compression include:

- Thorough explanation of the examination to ensure that the patient understands the need for compression
- Applying compression in a slow gentle manner while guiding the anatomy into position
- Establishing good rapport with the patient
- Scheduling examinations when the breast is least sensitive during the menstrual cycle
- Medicating patients with chronic breast sensitivity

PATIENT HISTORY

The needs of the individual patient are best satisfied when detailed personal and clinical histories are obtained.

Personal Data

Personal data that must be included in the mammography records consist of but are not limited to the following:

- Personal breast history to include familial and personal breast cancer risks
- Personal hormonal history that notes the onset of menses and onset of menopause
- History and type of hormone replacement therapy
- Gynecologic/reproductive history to include number of children and age of the patient at delivery

Clinical Data

Clinical data that should be included on mammography records consist of but are not limited to the following:

- Prior breast surgical history: site and type should be noted
- History of prior radiation therapy or other cancer treatment
- Documentation of prior mammograms
- Record of all breast pathologies to include location, size, and specific type (if known)
- Account of any prior breast procedures (aspiration, ultrasound, biopsy, etc.)
- Properly documented diagram of previous information on the clinical history sheet

BREAST SELF-EXAMINATION (BSE)

Breast self-examination is the single greatest support to mammographic examination.

Examination Positions

Erect (e.g., in the shower):   easiest and reliable for most women

Supine (e.g., in the bathtub): usually easier for large-breasted women

Important Points

- BSE should be done monthly, starting at age 20 years.
- Yearly breast examinations by a health care professional should be performed for women older than age 40 years; women younger than 40 should have a health care professional complete a breast examination every 3 years.
- Use the pads of the fingers.
- To become fully acquainted with the breast, explore them throughout the month and note how diet and hormones influence them.

Examination

- Recognize that fear perpetuates nonexamination.
- BSE is intended to find any breast changes that may lead to or hide pathology.
- Postmenopausal women should perform BSE on the same date each month.
- Premenopausal women should perform BSE at the beginning of (directly after menstruation) the menstrual cycle.
- Put the arm of the side to be examined behind the head (allows for breast tissue in the armpit to shift over the chest wall).
- Note the texture of the breast tissue (most breasts are lumpy).
- Note any rib abnormalities.
- Tissue in the axilla usually changes during the menstrual cycle.

Instructions for Proper BSE

1. Stand upright; using a mirror, view breasts for symmetry and skin deviations or discoloration (no two breasts are symmetrical)
2. Using one of the positions mentioned above, examine the breast using either the vertical strip or wedge pattern
3. It is important that the search is systematic and includes all breast tissue, especially the area of the axilla
4. The nipple should be gently squeezed to note any discharge; in some women, discharge may be normal
5. Note any "abnormal" lumps, their position and size

6. The steps should be repeated in both the upright and supine positions to ensure that all areas of the breast are thoroughly examined

HEALTH GUIDELINES

Clinical Evaluations

- Breast examinations by a health care professional should be performed every year for women older than 40 years; women younger than 40 should have a health care professional complete a breast examination every 3 years
- Mammography examinations:
  - Baseline: age 35–40 years
  - Every other year: age 40–49 years
  - Annually: age 50+ years

Unchangeable Risk Factors

Gender:	Women are 100 times more likely than men to develop breast cancer
Aging:	Breast cancer risk increases with age
Genetic Factors:	Approximately 5–10% cases of breast cancer can be attributed to inherited gene mutations
Family History:	Risk doubles if one first-degree (mother, daughter, or sister) relative has breast cancer; the risk increases five times if two first-degree relatives have the disease
Personal History:	A person with a history of cancer in one breast has a three to four times greater chance of developing cancer in the other breast
Race:	European-American women are more likely to acquire breast cancer, but Asian-American and African-American women are more likely to die from breast cancer
Previous Radiation:	Women who have had previous irradiation in the chest area have a slightly increased risk of developing breast cancer

Menstruation: Women who started menstruation early (before age 12) or menopause late (after age 50) have a *slightly* higher risk of developing breast cancer

Lifestyle-Related Risk Factors

Having Children: No children or first child after age 30 may slightly increase risk

Abortion: Induced or spontaneous abortions have not been proven to increase risk

Estrogen: Estrogen replacement therapy (ERT) may increase the risk with long-term use; risk returns to "normal" levels within 5 years of stopping ERT

Alcohol: Consumption of alcohol has been clearly linked to increased risk of breast cancer; two to five drinks each day increase the risk 1.5 times

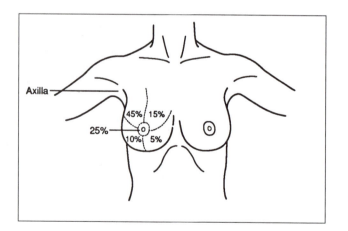

FIGURE 1-2

Breast cancer distribution by quadrant.

CHAPTER 2

Technical Proficiency Criteria

PROPER TECHNICAL FACTORS

Focal Spot

The most common focal spot sizes used in conventional mammography tubes range from 0.3 for small to 0.6 for large. Magnification mammography requires a focal spot size of at least 0.15.

Milliamperage

Generators with the highest milliampere output using the lowest milliampere station allow for the highest quality image. Recent improvements in x-ray generators allow for increased output. With small milliampere stations, longer time is often required, which may result in patient motion and a loss of resolution when using film that has little latitude.

The most commonly used milliampere stations are those with a large focal spot of 100 and a small focal spot of 15.

Kilovoltage

The kilovoltage used in mammography is relatively low and thus produces mammograms with high scale contrast. The kilovotltage setting depends primarily on the manufacturer's settings, the radiologist's preference, and target type. Most mammography units will allow for small incremental changes in the kilovoltage (1 kVp). The range of kilovoltage used in mammography is 23–30 kVp, with an average of 26 kVp.

Distance

Source-to-image distance (SID) should be kept at a maximum, especially when preforming magnification images. Long SID allows for better resolution. The SID receptor may range from 45 to 80 cm, with an average SID of at least 60 cm.

Grids

Either the stationary or reciprocating bucky may be used in mammography. Using a grid requires that the technical factors be increased an average of 2.5 times; however, this requirement should not be interpreted as an increase of 2.5 times the patient dose from nongrid exposures. Common grid ratios used in mammography are usually either 3.5:1 or 5:1, with a frequency of 30–72 lines per centimeter.

Magnification

The most common rate at which magnification views are accomplished is 1.5×. Other magnification rates range from 1.6× (to 2.0×). Magnification views should be performed with the smallest focal spot at the greatest distance and without a grid. The following are some of the most common reasons for using the magnification method:

- Outline characteristics of masses and microcalcifications
- Better visualization of tissues in dense breasts
- Evaluate surgical sites and assess borders
- Assess surgical specimens

BASIC TISSUE TYPES

Breast tissue is divided into three basic types: glandular, fibrous, and adipose. Breast type is generally classified by the amount of fibroglandular versus adipose tissue.

Fibroglandular

This tissue type is most common in women ages 15–30 years and in childless women older than age 30 years. Pregnant and lactating women also present with fibroglandular breasts. This tissue is usually the most difficult to penetrate mammographically because of the dense composition with very little fatty tissue.

Fibrofatty

This tissue type is most common in women ages 30–50 years and in younger women with multiple pregnancies. This type is easier to penetrate mammographically because the composition of the breast is half adipose and half fibroglandular.

Fatty

This tissue type is most common in postmenopausal women older than age 50 years. The breasts are atrophic, with minimal tissue density. The high fatty composition makes them easy to penetrate radiographically. Children, men, and prepubescent girls usually have this tissue classification.

ESSENTIAL IMAGING EVALUATION

Image Identification

Current regulations of the Federal Drug Administration (FDA) require that all mammograms be identified with the following permanent markings:

Patient name and any one of the following data: date of birth, medical record number, or any additional identifier

Date of examination

View/projection and laterality (specific breast), which should be marked near the axilla

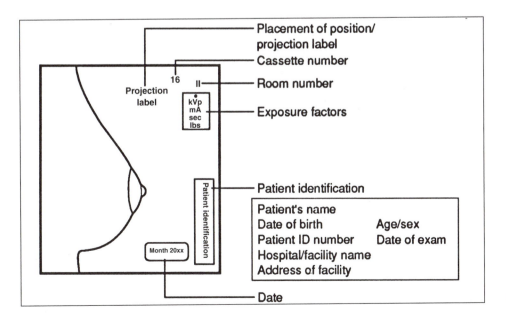

FIGURE 2-1

Name and location of the facility and the mammographer's specific identification markers

Cassette/screen identification and the specific mammography unit identifier if the facility has more than one mammography unit

Record and Report Results

Current FDA regulations require that all mammography reports include the following data within the written summary:

Patient name and any of the following: date of birth, medical record number, or any additional identifier

Date of examination and name of interpreting physician

Overall evaluation of the findings classified into one of the following categories: negative, benign, probably benign, suspicious, highly suggestive for malignancy, or incomplete

Clinical recommendations for future action, no matter what the diagnosis

Mediolateral Oblique

The mediolateral oblique view should demonstrate the pectoralis muscle to the level of the nipple. The intramammary fold should be illustrated with the nipple in profile. It is also imperative that the image of the breast tissue is not sacrificed to demonstrate the nipple in profile. The axillary portion of the breast should be clearly visible on the mediolateral oblique projection.

Craniocaudal Projection

The craniocaudal projection primarily demonstrates the medial, subareolar, central, and a portion of the lateral tissue of the breast. The primary portion demonstrated is the medial aspect of the breast. The nipple should be in profile. Minimal demonstration of the pectoralis muscle of the breast may be evident.

90° Lateral Projection

The 90° lateral projection should show the location of lesions, especially in the medial aspect of the breast. It is also used to demonstrate air–fluid levels or lesions. The straight lateral projection allows for a short SID when the side of interest is positioned closest to the film.

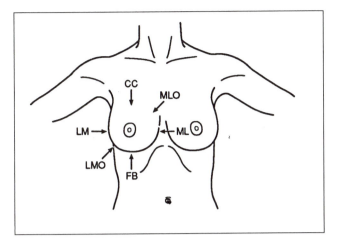

FIGURE 2-2

Exaggerated Craniocaudal Projection

The exaggerated craniocaudal projection is used to visualize deep lesions in the outer aspect of the breast to include most of the axillary tail.

Cleavage View

The cleavage view demonstrates the lesion in the posteromedial portion of the breast. All medial tissue of both breasts should be pulled anteriorly and visualized. Manual technical factors should be used.

Axillary Tail View

The axillary tail view is used to demonstrate the axillary portion of the breast, which includes most of the lateral aspect of the breast. The axillary tail should be in contact with the bucky.

Tangential View

The tangential view is used when demonstration of lesions closest to the skin surface is required. It is imperative that the palpable lesion be marked with a lead skin marker. It may be necessary to manually set the technical factors for the tangential projection.

CHAPTER 3

Position Proficiency Criteria

STANDARD VIEWS

Basic Principles

- The moveable margins of the breast are the lateral and inferior margins.
- The mobile tissues should be moved toward those immobile margins to maximize tissue visualization on the radiograph.
- Never move compression against a fixed margin or tissue.

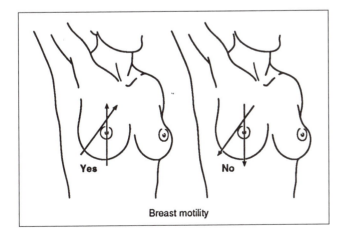

Breast motility

FIGURE 3-1

Craniocaudal

PURPOSE

The purpose of the craniocaudal position is to demonstrate all medial tissue and as much lateral tissue as possible.

Imaging Considerations

Better management in positioning can be obtained if the mammographer positions to the medial or opposite site of the breast being imaged.

To aid in relaxation of the patient's shoulder, the mammographer should place her hand on the shoulder of the side being imaged.

Optimum compression and tissue evaluation will be achieved if the patient is relaxed and understands the positioning criteria.

PROCEDURE

1. The patient should be parallel to the image receptor, with the head turned toward the unaffected breast.
2. The tube and bucky assembly should be perpendicular to the breast being imaged, with the tube angle at 0°.

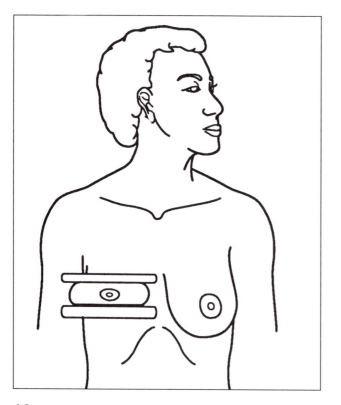

FIGURE 3-2

3. The patient should be as close to the image receptor as possible, with the outer edge of the receptor as close to the patient's chest wall as possible.

4. The patient should be leaning toward the receptor and holding onto the handlebar with the hand opposite the side being imaged.

5. The technologist should lift the breast, raising the inframammary fold (IMF) to its highest natural point.

6. The technologist should then raise the bucky to meet the IMF edge. The distance may range from 2 to 8 cm, depending on the mobility and elasticity of the tissue.

7. The breast is then placed atop the image receptor.

8. The technologist should, using both hands, delicately pull the lateral breast tissue forward, including as much as possible in the field.

9. The nipple should be in profile, with the breast directly over the center of the image receptor.

10. The technologist should check the height of the breast both medially and laterally before applying compression.

11. The mammographer should place the medial aspect of the opposite breast over the lateral corner of the image receptor, ensuring that the medial portion of the breast being imaged is included.

12. The technologist should apply compression slowly while holding the breast in position.

13. The mammographer should apply compression at least until the skin is taut or until optimal compression is achieved.

14. The patient should be instructed to relax the arm, specifically the humerus of the side being imaged.

15. The mammographer should instruct the patient to remain still and hold her breath during the exposure.

Mediolateral Oblique

PURPOSE

The purpose of the mediolateral oblique view is to demonstrate the anatomy of the upper outer breast quadrant. The properly positioned mediolateral oblique view will demonstrate more breast tissue than any other view.

Imaging Considerations

The image receptor must be parallel to the pectoralis muscle, which requires a 30–60° angle for most patients.

Tall thin patients usually require more tube angle, whereas short heavy patients require less angle to obtain an optimum film.

The more parallel the pectoralis muscle and the image receptor, the greater the amount of tissue included in the image.

PROCEDURE

1. The patient's pectoralis muscle should be parallel to the image receptor, which will require a 30–60° tube angle.
2. Using the principles of tissue mobility, the breast should be lifted medially, thereby ensuring that all breast tissue is in front of the image receptor.
3. The arm of the breast being imaged should grasp the handle.
4. The patient should be positioned close to the image receptor, with the superior lateral corner of the receptor fitting into the patient's axilla.
5. The humerus and elbow are draped over the superior portion of the image receptor. Flexion of the elbow will aid in relaxation of the pectoralis muscle.
6. The technologist should lift the breast away from the chest wall.
7. While turning the patient toward the image receptor, the breast is placed atop the image receptor.
8. The mammographer must ensure that the breast tissue has been lifted medially and that the position is maintained while placing the breast upon the receptor. Failure to do so will result in loss of tissue depiction.
9. The mammographer should begin applying compression while maintaining the position of the breast with a flat hand.
10. As compression is applied, the hand should be moved superiorly and medially to ensure that correct positioning is sustained.

11. The mammographer should apply compression at least until the skin is taut or until optimal compression is achieved.

12. To reduce the inframammary fold, the abdominal tissue at the inferior medial corner of the image receptor should be eased out of the field without affecting the tissue of the breast.

13. The mammographer should instruct the patient to remain still and hold her breath while the exposure is made.

ADDITIONAL PROJECTIONS

Axillary Tail

PURPOSE

The purpose of the axillary tail view is to demonstrate the tissue in the tail and in the upper outer portion of the breast. This projection may also be termed the Cleopatra view.

Imaging Considerations

There are two options when performing the axillary tail view.

The first is to simply oblique the patient anteriorly by placing the tail of the breast to the center of the image receptor. The image receptor is in the same position as that used for the craniocaudal projection.

The second option requires the mammographer to rotate the tube while keeping the image receptor parallel with the floor. The patient is then asked to lie back on the image receptor, as in the Cleopatra view.

PROCEDURE

1. If the patient does not have the mobility to tolerate the positioning without angling the tube, the tube should be rotated 10–30° medially and the beam should be perpendicular to the axillary tail.
2. The patient should be facing the image receptor.
3. The breast should be positioned in front of the image receptor by leaning the patient back onto the bucky.
4. All axillary breast tissue should be anterior to the image receptor.
5. The arm on the same side as the breast being imaged should grasp the handle and rest atop the image receptor, with the elbow relaxed.
6. The patient should be positioned so that the central ray enters midway between the nipple and axilla.
7. The mammographer should apply compression at least until the skin is taut or until optimal compression is achieved.
8. It may be necessary to increase the technical factors if the compression is not optimal due to the denseness of the area.
9. The mammographer should instruct the patient to remain still and hold her breath while the exposure is made.

Cleavage View

Purpose

The purpose of the cleavage view is to demonstrate lesions in the medial portion of the breast. The projection may also be termed the medial view, valley view, or double breast compression view.

Imaging Considerations

Special care should be taken to evaluate the inframammary folds and ensure that the folds meet the level of the image receptor.

The manual technique may more adequately penetrate the breast tissue.

The technologist may position from either behind or at the side of the patient.

Procedure

1. The patient is positioned in a way similar to that for the craniocaudal projection.
2. The breasts should be elevated and the image receptor raised to the level of the inframammary fold.
3. The medial portion of the breast being imaged should be placed in the center of the image receptor. This requires that both breasts be atop the receptor.
4. The patient's head must be turned away from the affected breast.
5. The arms are most comfortable if wrapped around the image receptor.

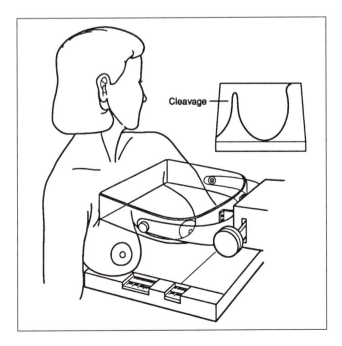

Cleavage

Figure 3-3

6. The patient should pull close to the film holder allowing for an increased amount of tissue to be placed on the receptor and for more secure positioning.

7. The mammographer should carefully apply compression to include as much medial tissue as possible. To do so, the technologist may have to manually draw the sternal tissue into the area while compressing.

8. The radiologist may request that compression not be used or that a spot compression device be used.

9. It may be necessary to increase the technical factors or use the manual set technique if the compression is not optimal due to the denseness of the area or the area of interest does not cover the ionization chamber.

10. The mammographer should instruct the patient to remain still and hold her breath while the exposure is made.

Exaggerated Craniocaudal

PURPOSE

The exaggerated craniocaudal projection is used to visualize the outer portion or axillary portion of the breast. This projection is especially helpful when imaging large breasts or lesions in the tail portion.

Imaging Considerations

The axillary tail is best visualized if the patient is rotated medially. The shoulder of the affected side must be relaxed to its lowest point to obtain the greatest amount of tissue.

PROCEDURE

1. The patient is positioned in a way similar to that for the craniocaudal projection.
2. The breasts should be elevated and the image receptor raised to the level of the inframammary fold.
3. The patient should be rotated medially 35–45°.
4. The lateral portion of the breast being imaged should be placed in the center of the image receptor.
5. The patient's head must be turned away from the affected breast.
6. The arms may be wrapped around the image receptor. The shoulder of the side being radiographed should be relaxed.
7. The tube should be angled approximately 5° laterally to avoid obstruction of the compression paddle by the humerus.
8. The mammographer should carefully apply compression and include as much lateral tissue as possible.
9. The technologist should draw as much lateral tissue as possible into the image while pressing back on the clavicle and applying compression.
10. The mammographer should instruct the patient to remain still and hold her breath while the exposure is made.

90° Mediolateral Projection

PURPOSE

This projection is used when two images must be taken at right angles from one another. This is common for localization of pathology or air–fluid demonstration.

Imaging Considerations

The imaging professional will note that the 90° mediolateral projection is performed more routinely than the 90° lateromedial projection because of ease in positioning. The lateral projection, which provides the least amount of OID in relation to the pathology of interest, should be done. The 90° mediolateral projection should be used when examining a lesion in the medial aspect of the breast.

PROCEDURE

1. The tube should be rotated 90° so that it is perpendicular to the breast.
2. The image receptor should be raised so that the superior outer edge of the image receptor fits into the patient's axilla.
3. The patient should be instructed to place her arm along the superior edge of the image receptor, with the outer edge of the receptor snug into the axilla.
4. The breast tissue should be moved superiorly and toward the midline.
5. The mammographer must ensure that all lateral breast tissue is in front of the image receptor. This requires that the breast be moved anteriorly.
6. The mammographer should carefully apply compression, and the patient should rotated, if necessary, to bring the breast into a true lateral position.
7. The compression should be applied until the breast tissue is taut. The compression device should be against the sternum or chest wall.
8. The ionization chamber should be directly over the mid-portion of the breast tissue.
9. The unaffected breast may need to be moved out of the image field. This may be accomplished by having the patient carefully pull it laterally, away from the chest wall with her hand.
10. The inframammary fold should be reduced by carefully pulling the abdominal tissue inferiorly.
11. The mammographer should instruct the patient to remain still and hold her breath while the exposure is made.

90° Lateromedial Projection

PURPOSE

This projection is used when two images must be taken at right angles from one another. This is common for localization of pathology or air–fluid demonstration.

Imaging Considerations

The lateral projection, which provides the least amount of OID in relation to the pathology of interest, should be done. Lesions in the medial aspect of the breast would require a 90° lateromedial projection.

PROCEDURE

1. The tube should be rotated 90° so that it is perpendicular to the breast.
2. The image receptor should be raised so that the entire outer edge of the image receptor is against the patient's sternum.
3. The patient should be instructed to raise her chin and place it on top of the image receptor, if possible.
4. The arm of the affected breast should be bent at the elbow, and the forearm should rest atop the image receptor.
5. The breast tissue should be moved superiorly and laterally.

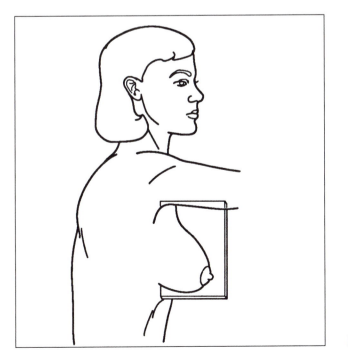

FIGURE 3-4

6. The mammographer must ensure that all medial breast tissue is parallel and against the image receptor.

7. The mammographer should carefully apply compression, and the patient should be rotated, if necessary, to bring the breast into a true lateral position.

8. The compression should be applied until the breast tissue is taut. The compression device should be against the latissimus dorsi.

9. The ionization chamber should be directly over the mid-portion of the breast tissue.

10. The unaffected breast should be behind the image receptor.

11. The inframammary fold should be reduced by carefully pulling the abdominal tissue inferiorly.

12. The mammographer should instruct the patient to remain still and hold her breath while the exposure is made.

Magnification Views

PURPOSE

The purposes of magnification views include but are not limited to the ability to differentiate between benign and malignant lesions by examination of the margins, evaluation of calcifications, and density of masses.

Magnification views may be accomplished with or without spot compression.

Imaging Considerations

The equipment requirements include the magnification platform and a tube with a focal spot of more than 0.2 mm. This focal spot size reduces geometric blurriness from the increased OID required for magnification images. No grid is used. Instead, the air-gap technique is employed, and long exposure times must be used.

PROCEDURE

1. The bucky should be removed, and the correct magnification platform should be attached to the mammography machine.
2. The patient should be informed that the exposure time will be increased and that suspended respiration is required for the entire exposure.
3. The portion if the breast tissue imaged will depend on the area of interest.
4. The area of interest will also determine the collimation and size of the compression device, if required.
5. The compression should be applied until the breast tissue is taut.
6. The mammographer should instruct the patient to remain still and hold her breath while the exposure is made.

Spot Images

PURPOSE

The spot view images are performed when suspicious areas are detected.

Imaging Considerations

Suspicious areas may be palpable or nonpalpable. Lesions may require the imaging professional to locate them by transferring measurements taken from the mammogram to the actual breast. The mammographer can use a BB, felt-tip skin marker, or X-spot to mark the area of interest.

Skilled mammographers may be able to position palpable masses without the use of an external landmark.

Manual technical factors may be employed to ensure proper penetration of tissue.

PROCEDURE

1. The focal compression device should be attached to the mammographic equipment. The type and size will depend on the area of suspicion and preference of the radiologist.

2. The patient should be informed that the exposure time will be increased and that suspended respiration will be required for the entire exposure.

FIGURE 3-5

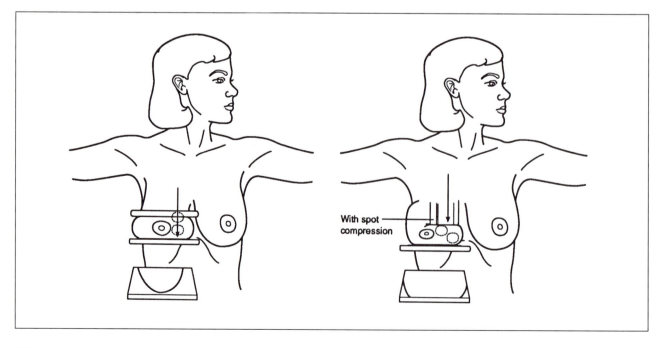

With spot compression

3. The collimation of the image will depend on the area of interest.

4. The lesion should be positioned with the central ray directly over the area of interest.

5. Nonpalpable lesions should be marked externally after localization from measurements derived from the mammogram.

6. Palpable lesions may be positioned by fingertip external localization.

7. The compression should be applied until the breast tissue is taut.

8. The mammographer should instruct the patient to remain still and hold her breath while the exposure is made.

Tangential Projection

PURPOSE

The purpose of the tangential projection is to evaluate suspected lesions located close to the skin surface.

Imaging Considerations

It is most common to use the manual technique when performing tangential views. It may be necessary to use a BB, felt-tip skin marker, or X-spot to mark the area of interest.

PROCEDURE

1. The focal compression device should be attached to the mammography equipment. The type and size will depend on the area of suspicion and preference of the radiologist.

2. The patient should be informed that the exposure time will be increased and that suspended respiration will be required for the entire exposure.

3. The collimation of the image will depend on the area of interest.

4. The lesion should be positioned with the central ray directly over the area of interest. Because the lesion is below the surface of the skin, the central ray will skim the surface of the breast.

5. The compression should be applied until the breast tissue is taut.

6. The mammographer should instruct the patient to remain still and hold her breath while the exposure is made.

MODIFIED STUDIES

Augmented Breast

PURPOSE

Augmented studies provide information by using positioning techniques that allow for better visualization of enhanced breast.

Imaging Considerations

It is important that the patient be completely informed of the necessary compression and displacement requirements when an implant is imaged. Technical factors must be set manually by the imaging professional.

The radiologist should inquire about the type of implant to evaluate mobility and compression ability. Mobility and compression ability will depend primarily on the following factors:

- Type of implant
- Degree of scarring and adhesion of the implant to the chest wall
- Breast size and amount of actual tissue

PROCEDURE

1. Positioning of the augmented breast should include the craniocaudal and mediolateral oblique projections. Technical factors should be manually set to ensure proper density of the implant.
2. The modified craniocaudal and mediolateral positions using the Eklund Method should also be performed.

FIGURE 3-6

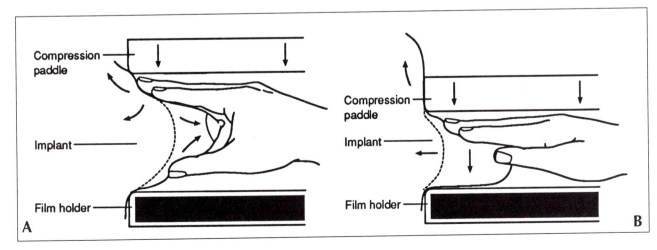

3. The Eklund Method has also been termed the "push back" because the implant is displaced superiorly and against the chest wall.

4. The modified craniocaudal view requires that the patient be positioned for the craniocaudal position with the following considerations:

   a. The breast tissue should be manipulated forward over the implant.

   b. The Eklund Method then requires the mammographer to press down gently on the breast with the fingertips and manipulate the implant back toward the chest wall.

   c. Compression should be carefully applied while securing the implant against the chest wall.

   d. The edge of the compression device should meet the superior edge of the implant by compressing the implant and free tissue.

   e. The mammographer should instruct the patient to remain still and hold her breath while the exposure is made.

5. The modified mediolateral oblique view requires that the patient be positioned for the mediolateral oblique position with the following alterations:

   a. The breast tissue is manipulated forward over the implant.

   b. The Eklund Method then requires that the mammographer press down gently on the breast with the fingertips and manipulates the implant back toward the chest wall.

   c. Compression should be carefully applied while securing the implant against the chest wall.

   d. The edge of the compression device should meet the superior edge of the implant by compressing the implant and free tissue.

   e. The mammographer should instruct the patient to remain still and hold her breath while the exposure is made.

Immobile Patient Positioning

PURPOSE

The purpose is modification of the standard projections for the patient confined to a gurney. Patients in wheelchairs can be imaged while in the wheelchair, but they may be imaged more easily if they are seated on a nonmovable bench.

Imaging Considerations

The following are modifications for each specific projection or view.

CRANIOCAUDAL

1. If performing the craniocaudal projection on a patient in the sitting position, the main consideration for the mammographer is to ensure that the patient leans into the image receptor. This will enable more breast tissue to be included in the mammogram.

2. When performing the craniocaudal projection on a patient on a gurney, it is important to lay the patient on the side opposite of the one to be radiographed.

3. The arm on the side down should be raised above the head, and the arm on the side of the affected breast should be placed by the patient's side.

4. The tube should be rotated so that it is perpendicular to the breast.

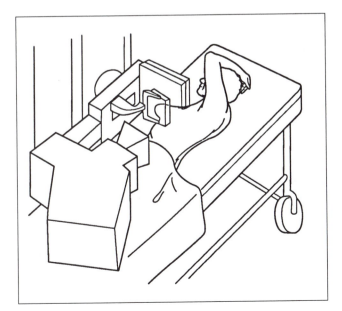

FIGURE 3-7

5. The image receptor should be perpendicular to the floor and the tube should be parallel to the floor.

6. Positioning is best done from behind the image receptor.

7. It is important that the image receptor be placed at the level of the inframammary fold when the breast is elevated.

8. The imaging professional will need to hold the patient's breast firmly against the image receptor while compressing the breast.

9. The opposite breast should be pulled away but may require that the medial portion rest on the edge of the film.

10. Compression should be applied until the breast is taut.

11. The mammographer should instruct the patient to remain still and hold her breath while the exposure is made.

MEDIOLATERAL OBLIQUE

1. If obtaining the mediolateral oblique view on a patient in the sitting position, the main consideration for the mammographer is to ensure that the patient leans into the image receptor. This will enable more breast tissue to be included in the mammogram. Two imaging professionals may need to assist in positioning.

2. When performing the mediolateral positioning on a patient on a gurney, it is important that the patient can tolerate elevation of the back of the gurney.

3. The patient will need to be placed between the image receptor and compression device.

4. The patient's pectoralis muscle should be parallel to the image receptor. This will require a 30–60° tube angle.

5. The image receptor should be placed against the patient's gurney.

6. Using the principles of tissue mobility, the breast should be lifted medially to ensure that all breast tissue is in front of the image receptor.

7. The patient should be positioned close to the image receptor, with the superior lateral corner of the receptor fitting into the patient's axilla.

8. The humerus and elbow are draped over the superior portion of the image receptor. Flexion of the elbow will aid in relaxation of the pectoralis muscle.

9. The technologist should lift the breast away from the chest wall.

10. The mammographer must ensure that the breast tissue has been lifted medially and that the position is maintained while placing the breast upon the receptor. Failure to do so will result in loss of tissue imaging.

11. Compression should be applied while holding the breast firmly in place and until the breast tissue is taut.

12. The mammographer should instruct the patient to remain still and hold her breath while the exposure is made.

LATEROMEDIAL

1. Lateromedial projections on a patient in the sitting position may be easier to obtain than mediolateral oblique projections.

2. It is imperative that the patient lean into the image receptor. This enables more tissue to be included on the image.

3. When performing the lateromedial positioning on a patient on a gurney, it important that the patient lay on her side. The breast of the up side will be radiographed.

4. The arms should be raised above the head, which is elevated on a pillow.

5. The tube should be rotated so that it is parallel with the gurney.

6. The image receptor should be between the breasts at the sternum, and the compression device should be at the outer margin of the breast against the rib cage.

7. The patient should be rolled slightly forward and the breast moved superior and laterally, with as much breast tissue as possible on the image receptor.

8. It is important that the pectoralis muscle be included on the image receptor.

9. The imaging professional should hold the patient's breast against the image receptor while compressing the breast.

10. The compression device should slide along the rib cage, and the inframammary fold will be included on the image.

11. Compression should be applied until the breast is taut.

12. The mammographer should instruct the patient to remain still and hold her breath while the exposure is made.

Positioning of the Large Breast

PURPOSE

To obtain similar quality films with modifications in positioning due to the breast size and body habitus of the patient.

Imaging Considerations

When obtaining mammograms on large-breasted patients, the following points should be considered when positioning the patient:

1. If the breast is too large to obtain all tissue on the craniocaudal projection with a large cassette, it may be necessary to acquire three separate mammograms for each breast.

2. If the breast is too large to obtain anterior tissue on the mediolateral oblique view, a separate mammogram should be taken specifically for the anterior tissue.

3. If uneven medial compression due to an overabundance of axillary tissue is present on the mediolateral oblique view, the mammographer should attempt the following:

   a. Reposition the patient to ensure that the superior corner of the image receptor is not buried too deep into the patient's axilla.

   b. Recheck the height and angle of the tube and receptor.

   c. Obtain two separate views, which may require separate tube angulation, of the lateral and medial tissue.

4. If the patient's abdomen protrudes, thus hindering the positioning of the inferior portion of the breast on the mediolateral oblique projection, it may be necessary for the imaging professional to modify positioning by using any or a combination of the following:

   a. Lean the patient into the image receptor.

   b. Reduce the angle of the tube and receptor to the minimal 30°. This will require the patient to lay back on the receptor.

   c. Using fingertips, gently push back the abdominal tissue while preserving the inframammary fold.

Positioning of the Small Breast

Purpose

To obtain similar quality films with modifications in positioning due to the breast size and body habitus of the patient.

Imaging Considerations

1. If the posterior tissue on the mediolateral oblique view is not imaged in its entirety, it may be necessary to increase the angle of the tube and receptor to a maximum of 70°.
2. If the mammographer is unable to visualize posterior tissue with the maximum angle, it may be necessary to use another position (exaggerated craniocaudal or 30° oblique position).
3. If the mammographer is unable to compress the tissue properly on the craniocaudal view, a rubber spatula can be used to compress and bring the tissue away from the chest wall while the compression device is engaged.

Postmastectomy Positioning

PURPOSE

The purpose of imaging the postmastectomy breast is to obtain images on the remaining tissue. The unaffected breast should also be imaged with the routine projections. Patients with unilateral breast cancer have a 50% risk increase of cancer development in the unaffected breast.

Imaging Considerations

Care should be taken to minimize discomfort, which may be more prevalent due to radiation treatment or postsurgical scarring.

The imaging professional should also be sensitive the feelings of the patient and her specific concerns regarding the mastectomy site and future cancer risk.

PROCEDURE

1. A mediolateral oblique projection of the mastectomy site should be performed. Positioning is similar to that of the routine mediolateral oblique.

2. An anteroposterior view of the axilla for evaluation of the lymph nodes and tissue should also be routinely performed on mastectomy sites.

3. The radiologist may also request spot view images of suspicious areas.

MAMMOGRAPHY OF THE MALE PATIENT

Caudocranial Projection

PURPOSE

The purpose of the caudocranial position is to demonstrate all medial tissue and the retroareolar area in profile.

Imaging Considerations

Gynecomastia is the most common breast pathology in men and is usually marked by an increase in fibroglandular tissue in the retroareolar area.

To aid in the relaxation of the patient's shoulder, the mammographer should place a hand on the shoulder of the side being imaged.

Optimum compression and tissue evaluation will be achieved if the patient is relaxed and understands the positioning criteria.

PROCEDURE

1. The tube should be rotated 180° so that the compression device is inferior and the image receptor superior.

2. The patient must face the tube and should be able to rest the arm on the side of the breast being imaged atop the image receptor.

3. The breast should be positioned so that the superior portion is touching the image receptor.

4. The patient can rest his chin on the image receptor and the arm on the side of the unaffected breast should be brought behind the patient's back.

5. Compression is accomplished by using the palm of the hand or a spatula to spread the tissue.

6. The compression should be applied until the breast tissue is taut.

7. The mammographer should instruct the patient to remain still and hold his breath while the exposure is made.

Mediolateral Oblique Projection

PURPOSE

The purpose of the mediolateral oblique view is to demonstrate the anatomy of the upper outer breast quadrant.

Imaging Considerations

The image receptor must be parallel to the pectoralis muscle, which on the male patient usually requires a 65–70° tube angle.

PROCEDURE

1. The patient's pectoralis muscle should be parallel to the image receptor. This will require at least a 65° tube angle.
2. The breast should be lifted medially, thereby ensuring that all breast tissue is in front of the image receptor.
3. The hand on the side of the breast being imaged should grasp the handle.
4. The patient should be positioned close to the image receptor, with the superior lateral corner of the receptor fitting into the patient's axilla anterior to the latissimus dorsi.
5. The humerus and elbow are draped over the superior portion of the image receptor. Flexion of the elbow will aid in relaxation of the pectoralis muscle.
6. The technologist should lift the breast away from the chest wall.
7. The mammographer should begin applying compression while maintaining the position of the breast with a flat hand.
8. As compression is applied, the hand should be moved superiorly and medially to ensure that correct positioning is sustained.
9. The superior edge of the compression paddle should be just inferior and medial to the head of the humerus.
10. The mammographer should apply compression at least until the skin is taut or until optimal compression is achieved.
11. Compressing the male breast may require the use of a rubber spatula to ensure that the breast is spread and held in place until the compression device is engaged.
12. To reduce the inframammary fold on a patients with a protruding abdomen, the abdominal tissue at the inferior medial corner of the image receptor should be eased out of the field without affecting the tissue of the breast.
13. The mammographer should instruct the patient to remain still and hold his breath while the exposure is made.

SPECIAL PROCEDURES

Needle Localization

PURPOSE

The purpose of needle localization is to determine the site of a lesion preoperatively. Precise needle placement is of the utmost importance. Procedural understanding by the patient is imperative.

Imaging Considerations

Methods of preoperative needle localization depend on the location of the lesion in the breast, surgical approach for removal, and patient condition.

The mammographer should explain the procedure to the patient and obtain proper consent. All preoperative needle placements should be done under sterile conditions. Sedation is contraindicated because the patient must be alert and able to follow instructions. The patient should never be left alone in the room. The technologist should be prepared for any reaction from the patient, including fainting.

Special equipment may include a paddle with coordinate measurements that has either a single or many holes along its edge to allow the needle to be placed into the breast.

PROCEDURE

The localization guides will depend on the radiologist's preference and the location of the lesion.

1. The introduction of the needle depends on the location of the lesion.

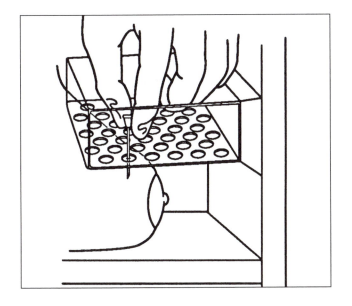

FIGURE 3-8

41

2. Measurements to determine needle placement should be done with the aid of craniocaudal and 90° lateral views.

3. The breast should remain compressed while these films are evaluated.

4. It may be necessary to use spot compression or magnification devices to evaluate and localize the lesion.

5. The approach is determined by the radiologist. The patient is usually in the sitting position.

6. Using the measurements and aperture compression device, the location of the lesion, with reference to that of the aperture, should be noted. The radiologist may want to mark the skin.

7. The needle may then be introduced, under sterile conditions, if the radiologist is satisfied with the localization from the previous radiographs.

8. A mammogram is then taken to evaluate the needle placement.

9. If the radiologist is satisfied with the view, compression should be released, making sure that the needle does not "catch" in the aperture of the compression device.

10. The unit is then repositioned 90° from the first view and recompressed, and an exposure is made.

11. The radiologist will evaluate both mammographic views for needle placement.

12. If it is the preference of the radiologist and surgeon, methylene blue dye may be injected at this point, with a small amount of air to use as localization in case the needle slips out of position.

13. The securing of the needle will depend on the size of the breast and the preference of the radiologist.

14. The hub may be removed and the needle secured, or the hub may be left on the needle as the needle is secured.

15. A piece of surgical mask cut to fit the breast contour or a small piece of paper drape may be used to secure the needle to the breast. Gauze is contraindicated because it may catch on the needle and dislodge it.

16. The films sent to the operating room should be marked in sequence and should include a breast diagram with the lesion position and the radiologist's contact number for the surgeon.

Ductography

PURPOSE

The purpose of the ductogram is to determine possible reasons for abnormal nipple discharge.

Imaging Considerations

Galactography is a term also used to denote this procedure. The duct expressing the fluid is cannulated. The procedure may be performed under ultrasound guidance. The patient must be informed as to the specifics of the procedure.

PROCEDURE

1. Routine scout views are taken of both breasts. Additional views of the affected breast may be required by the radiologist.
2. The patient may be in either an oblique recumbent or recumbent position, with the arm on the side of the affected breast behind the patient's head.
3. The radiologist may use a bright lamp focused on the nipple area.
4. The area should be cleaned with aseptic solution.
5. The radiologist, patient, or imaging professional, with a radial motion, will attempt to express fluid from the suspicious duct.
6. Once identified, the radiologist will cannulate the duct of interest. The type of cannula is determined by the radiologist.
7. Dilation of the duct can be achieved by using galactographic dilators, if necessary.
8. Once the cannula is introduced into the duct, the patient should be positioned in the mammography machine.
9. Magnification views are usually taken from the craniocaudal and 90° lateral projections after contrast material has been injected.
10. Addition images with or without magnification may be necessary to visualize filling defects and lesions.
11. It is suggested that lesions being localized for surgical resection be injected with a methylene blue dye and contrast mixture.

Fine-Needle Aspiration

PURPOSE

Fine-needle aspiration is performed to obtain a specimen for cytologic analysis. It is an aid used to differentiate between benign and malignant lesions in both symptomatic and asymptomatic patients.

Imaging Considerations

It is important that the procedure be explained clearly to the patient. The needle should remain in the breast for only a few seconds. The procedure usually does not call for the use of anesthesia, although the radiologist may employ an anesthesia.

PROCEDURE

1. Routine scout views are taken of both breasts. Additional views of the affected breast may be required by the radiologist.
2. The patient may be in either an oblique recumbent or a recumbent position, with the arm on the side of the affected breast behind the patient's head.
3. The lesion should be palpated and localized. To prevent movement of the mass when inserting the needle, the skin should be spread tightly over the lesion.

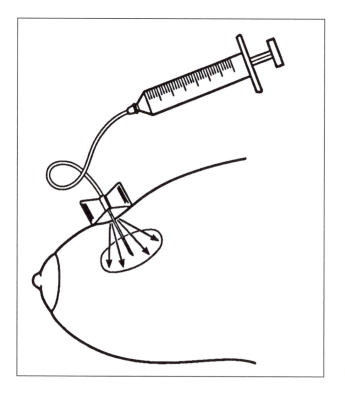

FIGURE 3-9

4. Using an aseptic technique, the area should be wiped with alcohol before the needle is inserted.

5. The use of a butterfly needle and syringe (20 cc) is employed. The mammographer should pull back on the plunger of the syringe as soon as the needle has entered the mass.

6. The radiologist will usually move the needle around in a circular motion to ensure that an adequate number of cells have been aspirated from the area.

7. The mammographer will then be instructed to slowly release the plunger portion of the syringe, and the radiologist will remove the needle.

8. Care should be taken not to release any cells from the needle because of the negative pressure in the syringe.

9. Direct pressure should be applied to the site with removal of the needle.

10. A cytology slide should be made and sent for evaluation.

Magnetic Resonance Imaging (MRI)

PURPOSE

MRI enables diagnosis of breast malignancy with a more sensitive and specific modality that conventional mammography.

Imaging Considerations

To use MRI rather than the conventional means of diagnosis in breast cancer detection, the MR equipment must meet certain standards. The MR unit must have high resolution and should make use of fat suppression to differentiate fat from tumors. Both criteria aid in the diagnosis between different tissue types. MRI is often used in cases in which abnormalities are denoted on a mammogram or in patients with breast implants, diagnosis of ruptured implants, or characterization between tissue types. In some instances, hormones directly influence tissue changes within the breast. Therefore, MRI should be performed within the first 2 weeks of the menstrual cycle.

In many cases, a contrast agent such as gadolinium-DTPA is used to aid in breast tissue enhancement. With the use of contrast material, benign lesions may be differentiated from malignant lesions. Tumors, for the most part, will employ rapid contrast enhancement within the first 5 min of contrast introduction. If contrast is used for the scan, both pre- and postgadolinium images must be obtained as part of the protocol.

Although MRI has many advantages, it has disadvantages. Disadvantages include high cost, inadequacy for the detection of microcalcifications, lesions found within the breast still must be biopsied, and the presence of respiratory and cardiac artifacts.

PROCEDURE

1. Explain the entire procedure, length of the procedure, and the atmosphere of the MR unit to the patient. Obtain the patient's consent for administering of contrast agent.

2. A marker that will be visible to MRI may be placed directly over the nipple and or any palpable areas within the breast of concern.

3. Introduce the contrast agent intravenously into the patient.

4. Place the patient prone on the table in the most comfortable position to minimize movement during and between scans for this lengthy study.

5. The breast of concern should be placed within the imaging breast coil.

6. Some coils enable breast compression, which would result in fewer slices to image the entire breast.

7. The patient is positioned in relation to the longitudinal and horizontal light beams where axial or sagittal slices may be obtained.

8. Contrast is introduced, and slices are scanned.

ANALYSIS

Imaging of the normal breast with contrast enhancement will enhance all vessels supplying the breast, with a slight increase of contrast uptake posterior to the nipple. Malignant disease such as ductal carcinoma in situ and lobular carcinoma in situ will enhance with contrast, whereas benign lesions do not typically enhance with contrast.

Ultrasound

PURPOSE

Ultrasound is most advantageous because of its ability to distinguish between solid and cystic lesions without the use of radiation. Ultrasound is also helpful in detecting symmetrical versus asymmetrical lesions within the breast.

Imaging Considerations

Ultrasound is a noninvasive way to visualize tissues and lesions within the breast through the use of sound waves. Sound waves are sent into the body by a transducer; the waves return to the transducer after they have contacted the tissue in its path. Ultrasound enables the sonographer to locate lesions within the breast, determine whether a lesion is solid or cystic, and differentiate between dense tissue types. By no means should ultrasound be used as a primary tool for diagnosing breast pathology; it should serve only as a supplemental tool to mammography. Ultrasound is not always able to detect the smallest lesions, evaluate the whole anatomy of the breast accurately, and is incapable of diagnosing changes in tissue density and breast contour the way conventional mammography can.

The disadvantages of sonography explain why it is not the primary modality for diagnosing breast cancer. Ultrasound is incapable of imaging the posterior portion of the breast and the tissue posterior to the nipple. Ultrasound is not able to detect microcalcifications. Sonography of the breast also involves careful analysis of the breast images by the sonographer to ensure a proper diagnosis. Results of the ultrasound depend on the sonographer and his/her ability to manipulate the transducer and interpret the images.

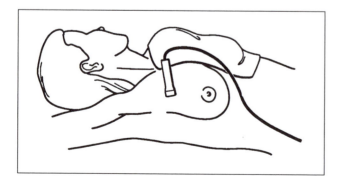

FIGURE 3-10

PROCEDURE

1. Explain the entire procedure to the patient. The procedure is noninvasive so written consent from the patient is not required.
2. Review the patient's mammogram to locate any highly suspicious areas that may require more concentration.
3. Place the patient supine on the sonography table, exposing the breast of interest.
4. The arm on the side of the breast being examined should be placed above the patient's head.
5. Ultrasound gel, which serves as the medium for the sound waves, is placed on the breast.
6. The breast will be scanned in a clockwise method to ensure that nothing is missed.
7. The breast will be scanned in two different planes: transverse and longitudinal.
8. If any lesions of concern are identified during the scan, measurements of the lesion are made in both planes. Documentation includes obtaining an image with measurements and locating the lesion on a schematic drawing of the breast.

ANALYSIS

Ultrasound is capable of distinguishing a solid mass from a cystic mass. A solid mass is identifiable by its smooth borders surrounding the lesion or mass and indicates that the mass is most likely benign. A solid mass with an irregular border surrounding the lesion or mass indicates possible malignancy. Sonography can also determine the nature of the fluid within the breast. If the lesion represents the true characteristics of a cyst, no further evaluation such as a biopsy is required. With sonography, sonographers are also capable of detecting any intracystic lesions, abscesses, or hematomas.

Stereotactic Breast Biopsy

PURPOSE

Stereotactic biopsy provides a special technique in which one is able to pinpoint a nonpalpable abnormality that is visualized on conventional mammography. Stereotactic biopsy uses digital radiography to visualize tissue with even better resolution. With digital mammography, the image of the breast is computerized and then recreated. The image created by a computer rather than through a photograph allows the radiologist to see specific areas of the breast and determine whether these areas are tissue tissue or fat.

Imaging Considerations

For patients who present with a probable benign lesion within the breast, a simple stereotactic procedure may eliminate the need for surgery. Mammograms, which demonstrate a probable malignant lesion, allow for confirmation of the diagnosis of malignancy before surgery is performed. The new technology of stereotactic breast biopsy provides several advantages to the patient: accuracy is similar to that of an excisional biopsy, discomfort and recovery time are reduced, no cosmetic defects result on the breast, cost is less, and radiation is minimized through digital imaging. Contraindications apply to patients who may be taking anticoagulants and to patients with severe back pain or arthritis, which inhibits the patient lying prone for an extended period.

Mammographers should obtain specialized training in this specialized technique to perform the advanced procedure competently and to aid the radiologist performing the biopsy.

FIGURE 3-11

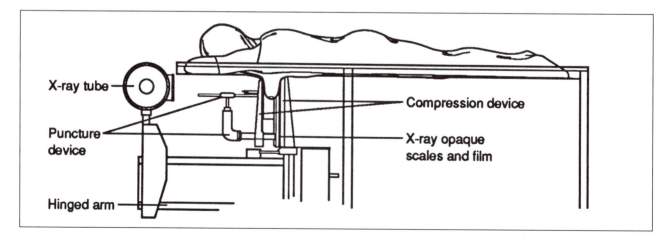

PROCEDURE

1. Explain the examination to the patient and obtain proper consent for the procedure.

2. The patient is placed prone on the stereotactic biopsy table. The breast of interest is suspended through the opening in the table.

3. Two digital radiographs are obtained of the breast from two different angles to pinpoint the location of the abnormality.

4. The computer properly calculates the angle and depth needed for proper needle placement.

5. The skin of the breast is prepared with a Betadine solution, and a sterile field is created.

6. A local anesthetic is administered.

7. A small incision at the entrance site for the needle is made with a surgical blade.

8. Manually advance the needle on the biopsy device to the exact location of the lesion by the coordinates calculated by the computer. The biopsy needle is a relatively large-gauge needle that consists of an inner needle with a trough and an overlying sheath. The needle is attached to the biopsy gun, which is spring loaded. When the gun is discharged, the inner portion of the needle projects forward, allowing the trough to fill with tissue, and the overlying sheath projects forward to cut the tissue and secure the trough of the needle. Rapid firing of the biopsy gun allows for minimal discomfort to the patient and a good tissue sample.

9. More than one biopsy may be taken.

10. Once a biopsy is taken, a specimen radiograph may be taken to evaluate the tissue removed. If the lesion appears to have been missed, coordinates should be recalculated and another attempt made.

11. Completion of the procedure requires pressure on the site of needle entrance to reduce the chance of a hematoma. Once bleeding has ceased, the incision is dressed and the patient is sent home. The patient should be instructed to avoid any strenuous activity for 24 h after the procedure.

12. Specimen tissue must be sent for analysis.

ANALYSIS

Once the final pathology has been determined, results must be compared with the original diagnosis made from the mammogram. If the pathology results are inconsistent with the mammogram diagnosis, the patient may be considered for an excisional biopsy. If lesions are found to be benign, patients are recommended to obtain a follow-up mammogram in 6 months to evaluate the stability of the lesion.

CHAPTER 4

Quality Control and Management Proficiency Criteria

Compression

Compression is used for reducing the thickness of the breast tissue, which is essential for the production of a high-quality mammogram. With compression, tissue thickness is decreased, which results in decreased patient dose and increased image contrast, quality, and sharpness. At the present time, all mammographic units must be equipped with a compression device, which allows mammographers to apply gentle pressure to the breast to obtain quality mammograms. However, because compression is applied for many examinations, it is essential to maintain image quality. Mammographers can ensure that adequate compression is maintained by testing both the manual adjustments and the powered mode. Most importantly, one can ensure that the equipment does not allow too much compression to be applied.

This test should be performed initially with any new equipment, semiannually, and when reduced compression is suspected.

PURPOSE

To evaluate and ensure that adequate compression is maintained through testing both the manual adjustment and the powered mode. Whether compression is checked through the powered mode or manual mode, the compression should meet a minimum of 25 lbs. and a maximum of 40 lbs. Most importantly, ensure that the equipment does not allow too much compression to be applied.

MATERIALS

> Flat bathroom scale
> Towels
> Mammographic unit

PROCEDURE

1. Place a towel on the cassette holder to protect it.
2. Place the bathroom scale on the towel, with the dial facing out for easy reading, and make sure that the center of the scale is located directly under the compression device.
3. Place one or more towels on top of the scale to protect the compression device.
4. Using the power drive, allow the compression device to compress until it stops automatically.
5. Read and record the compression in pounds and then release the compression.
6. Using the manual drive, move the compression device down until it cannot compress any more.
7. Read and record the compression in pounds and then release the compression.

ANALYSIS

To evaluate adequate compression in the power drive mode, the compression should range anywhere from 25 to 40 lbs. to be within acceptable limits. To evaluate the compression under manual drive, compression of at least 25 lbs. should be achievable, and compressions up to 40 lbs. are acceptable.

If the test fails to meet these criteria, a service engineer should be contacted to make the appropriate internal adjustments.

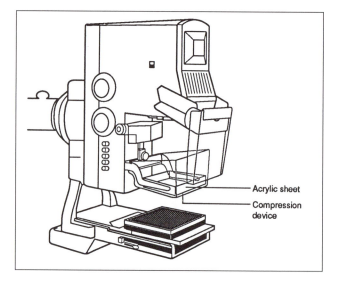

Acrylic sheet
Compression device

FIGURE 4-1

Darkroom Cleanliness

Minimizing artifacts that mimic microcalcification begins with and depends on darkroom cleanliness. Mammographic images reflect on how well the darkroom is maintained. Darkrooms must be maintained with a daily cleaning of the countertops, processor feed trays, pass boxes, floors, and a weekly cleaning of air vents and safelights. Construction of the darkroom is also an important factor that must be kept in mind. It is important that neither heating nor air-conditioning vents are installed above the countertops or the processor feed trays. Ceilings should be constructed of a solid material to reduce any dust or other particles from falling on work surfaces. Storage space or cabinets should not be installed above the countertops because these are spaces where dust may accumulate.

This test should be performed daily before patients are seen.

PURPOSE

To minimize image artifacts that may cause misdiagnosis.

MATERIALS

Wet mop and pail
Lint-free towels

PROCEDURE

1. Damp mop the floor (daily) and walls (weekly) if dust is a problem.
2. Remove all items from the countertop and work areas.
3. With a clean damp towel, wipe the countertops, processor feed trays, and the inside of the pass boxes. *Make sure that your hands remain clean.*
4. Once a week, either wipe off or vacuum the overhead air vents and safelights. Remember to do this before proceeding with the daily routine cleaning of the darkroom.

ANALYSIS

Darkroom cleanliness is evaluated best by screen cleanliness. Evaluate films for dust and dirt artifacts that appear on mammographic images.

Darkroom Fog

Every darkroom should be inspected for darkroom fog on a regular basis to ensure that outside light sources or the safelighting within the room are not fogging the mammographic film. During this inspection, it is important to evaluate all safelights to ensure proper mounting of the appropriate distance from the work space. Also, ensure that safelight filters are not cracked. Cracked safelights or other sources of white-light leaks result in the fogging of film, which decreases the contrast of a piece of film, which creates differences in densities between one film and the next. Different sheets of film may demonstrate more or less density depending on the amount of fog exposure.

This test should be performed initially and at least semiannually thereafter. This test should also be performed when safe-light bulbs or filters are changed or whenever fog may be suspected.

PURPOSE

The purpose is to evaluate and ensure that the mammographic film is not exposed to any fogging light sources inside or outside of the darkroom.

MATERIALS

Densitometer

Mammographic film (from an unopened box)

Opaque card

Watch

PROCEDURE

1. Check that the safe-light bulb wattage is correct and make sure that the filters do not appear cracked or faded.

2. Check for the correct distance between the safelight and the countertops.

3. Turn off all the lights in the darkroom. Before beginning, allow 5 min to pass so the eyes can adjust.

4. Inspect the darkroom for any obvious light leaks that may be occurring. Check around the doors, pass boxes, processors, and the ceiling. When checking for light leaks, evaluate for leaks from different aspects of the room to ensure that the inspection is thorough.

5. Fix any and all light leaks before proceeding with the test.

6. Check for any afterglow that may be occurring with the darkroom's overhead fluorescent lights by turning the lights on for 2 min and then turning them off.

7. Load a cassette with the appropriate film in total darkness.

8. Exit the darkroom and make an exposure with the phantom. Place the phantom on the cassette holder and make sure that the phantom is lined up with the evenly with the chest wall side of the cassette.

9. Bring compression down atop the phantom.

10. Either set the manual exposure time in milliamperes or place the phototimer sensor in the appropriate position to match all previous tests for a 4–4.5-cm compressed breast. Consistency is very important.

11. Return to the darkroom, remove the exposed film, and lay it on the counter with the emulsion side facing up. Cover one-half of the phantom image with the opaque card so the card is perpendicular to the chest wall edge of the film.

12. With the safelights on, allow the film to lay on the countertop for 2 min.

13. Process the film.

14. After the film is processed, use the densitometer to measure close to the dividing edge, which separates the fogged from the unfogged portion of the phantom. When measuring with the densitometer, try not to measure close to any test objects within the phantom.

15. In a similar manner, measure the density of the fogged portion against the unfogged portion. When obtaining this measurement, be sure to place the densitometer at a spot adjacent to these portions across the boundary of the opaque card.

16. Determine the amount of fog by subtracting the density of the unfogged portion from that of the fogged portion of the phantom.

ANALYSIS

The density difference obtained from the last step of the procedure should not be greater than 0.05. If the density difference is greater, there must be an evident source of fog that must be determined and corrected. Re-examine the darkroom for any light leaks, safelight imperfections, and the correct safelight bulb wattage. This test indicates the length of time a film may be "safe" within the darkroom.

Film–Screen Contact

Mammography requires a consistent level of quality to be maintained. In any modality but especially mammography, film–screen contact must be maintained for purposes of detail and spatial resolution. Film–screen contact significantly affects the image sharpness. In mammography, film–screen systems have a higher spatial resolution of 16–20 cycles/mm as opposed to only 4–8 cycles/mm for conventional systems. However, to maintain either level of resolution, the film and the screen must remain in the closest possible contact with one another.

This test should be performed initially with any new cassette. Cassettes should also be evaluated semiannually and anytime thereafter when decreased image sharpess is suspected.

PURPOSE

To ensure that all mammographic cassettes are producing the highest image quality by ensuring that proper film–screen contact is occurring.

MATERIALS

Copper screen mesh consisting of 40 wires per inch

Acrylic sheets 4 cm thick to ensure a reasonable exposure time

Densitometer

All screens and cassettes to be tested

Mammographic film

PROCEDURE

1. Begin by carefully cleaning all the screens and cassettes with a screen cleaner. Be sure that the insides of the cassettes are cleaned thoroughly.

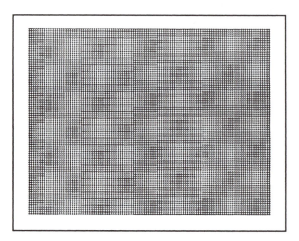

FIGURE 4-2

2. Allow the insides of the screens to air dry for approximately 30 min before closing or loading the cassettes with film.

3. Load all the cassettes with the appropriate film size.

4. Allow the cassettes to sit for 15 min so that any air trapped within the cassettes can escape.

5. One at a time, lay the cassettes atop the cassette holder (bucky/grid). Do not use the grid for this test.

6. Place the wire mesh directly on top of the cassette so that it is centered with reference to the cassette.

7. Place the acrylic sheet (only if needed) on top of the compression paddle and then raise the compression paddle and position it close the tube port. The acrylic sheet is used to ensure an exposure time of at least 0.5 sec and to produce an optical density of 0.70–0.80 over the area of the mesh nearest the chest wall side of the film. The acrylic sheet will also aid in minimizing the amount of scatter radiation reaching the film.

8. Select a manual technique setting that will provide an optical film density of 0.70–0.80 nearest the chest wall edge of the radiograph. Use 25–28 kVp.

9. Expose and process the film.

10. Continue to repeat these first nine steps on each cassette to be tested.

11. Hang the exposed radiographs on the view box and stand back at least 3 ft to evaluate. During the evaluation, look for any areas that appear "blurry" or even dark. One or the other of these signs indicates areas of poor film–screen contact.

ANALYSIS

Areas on the films representing poor film–screen contact and measure more than 1 cm in diameter should be retested. The entire procedure should be repeated, beginning with cleaning the screen and the cassette. Once the cassette has been retested and the large area of poor film–screen contact has not been eliminated, this cassette should be replaced. Films with multiple areas of poor film–screen contact that measure less than 1 cm in diameter are still within acceptable limits. Often the darkened areas that measure less than 1 cm represent poor screen cleaning and are signs of dirt or dust. Poor film–screen contact can also result from damaged cassettes, deterioration of foam within the cassette, which does not allow for sufficient equalized pressure, or air trapped within the cassette.

Fixer Retention

Fixer ingredients allow for silver halide crystals to be removed from the film. This agent is affected by silver recovery and replenishment rates. If fixing agents are not removed from the film in the wash cycle; a yellowing or tarnishing of the film may be evident. This yellowing is due to a chemical reaction between thiosulfate and silver in the emulsion producing silver sulfide, which is responsible for the staining of the image.

This test should be performed quarterly. The American National Standards Institute recommends that the acceptable limit of residual hypo be less than 2 μg/cm^2 for diagnostic radiography and 5 μm/cm^2 for mammography.

PURPOSE

The purpose of the fixer retention test is to evaluate the quantity of residual fixer in a processed film.

MATERIALS

A commercial hypo retention kit may be purchased

To make your own kit, use the following ingredients, which can be obtained from a photographic supply store: 75 mL distilled water, 12.5 mL 28% acetic acid, and 0.75 g silver nitrate. Stir the distilled water and acetic acid together, add silver nitrate while stirring, and continue to stir until all is dissolved. To this solution, add enough distilled water to create a solution of 100 mL. Store in a dark container in a cool dark place.

Hypo indicator strip (if not using kit)

8 × 10 film

Processor

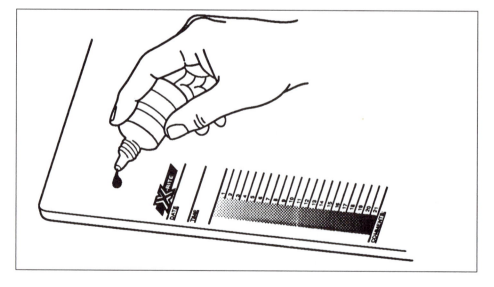

FIGURE 4-3

PROCEDURE

1. Remove the film directly from the film bin and process.
2. After film has been processed, place one drop of hypo test solution on the film.
   a. If using single emulsion film, the solution should be placed on the emulsion side.
   b. If using dual emulsion film, each side must be tested individually. Solution should be placed so that it does not interfere with the area being tested on the opposite side.
3. Allow the solution to stand for 2 min.
4. Excess solution should be removed by blotting with a cloth. Do not rub.
5. Place stained area over a white sheet of paper and lay the hypo indicator strip so a comparative analysis can be done.
6. Analysis should be done immediately because light will cause the stain to darken.

ANALYSIS

If the test indicates that levels are not within the guidelines, repeat the test immediately. If similar test results are obtained, corrective measures should be taken. Troubleshooting measures may include evaluating:

1. The wash tank to ensure that it contains the correct water levels
2. The wash water flow rate to ensure that it is set to the manufacturer's guidelines
3. The fixer replenishment rate to ensure that it is set to the manufacturer's guidelines.

If all appears to be correct, the processor may not be the problem. Consult the film manufacturer for possible suggestions.

Phantom Imaging

Phantom imaging is one of the most important factors of mammography quality assurance. Performance of the test allows for evaluation of resolution, contrast, density changes, uniformity, and possible tube degeneration. By using a phantom, the output of the mammography unit can be evaluated over time and many units may be maintained.

This test should be performed initially after equipment calibration. To establish a baseline level, the processor should be filled with fresh chemistry at the time the equipment is calibrated. Once the baseline is achieved, the phantom testing should be performed at least monthly or anytime the equipment (processors or units) is serviced or when fluctuation of image quality is suspected.

PURPOSE

To establish a baseline of quality that allows for evaluation of the equipment involved with the entire imaging chain over time, to ensure that the equipment is functioning properly, and to maintain the highest level of quality achievable.

MATERIALS

Mammography-accredited phantom: a square acrylic block filled with a variety of simulated masses, fibers, and specks and is the equivalent a 4–4.5-cm compressed breast)

Acrylic disk: a disk 1 cm in diameter and 4 mm thick that serves primarily to create a density difference

Mammographic cassette loaded with film

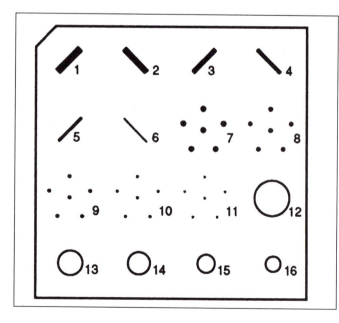

FIGURE 4-4

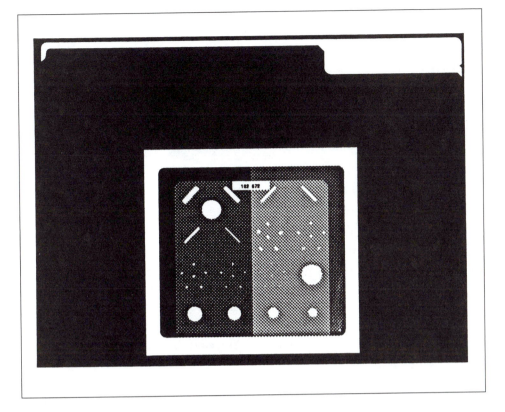

FIGURE 4-5

Original phantom image

Previous phantom image

Densitometer

Control charts

Magnifying lens

PROCEDURE

1. Position the loaded cassette in the cassette holder of the bucky.

2. Secure the 4-mm-thick acrylic disk on the phantom consistent with its placement on all previous phantom films taken. It is important to place the acrylic disk in an area on the phantom that does not interfere with any of details of the phantom. *Suggestion: Secure the acrylic disk to the phantom with glue so consistent location is achieved.*

3. Place the phantom on the bucky, aligning the edge of the phantom with the chest wall side of the image receptor. Position the phantom as if it were a breast. *Note: On the phantom, there is a small indention resembling the location of nipple, so make sure that this nipple marker is positioned away from the chest wall side of the image receptor.*

4. Lower the compression device to bring the paddle in contact with the phantom.

5. Prepare to make the exposure, which should resemble the outcome of a 4–4.5-cm compressed breast. This may be done in either of two ways:

   a. If AEC is used, ensure that the phototimer detector is positioned under the phantom but is consistent in location with all previous phantom images.

   b. If the manual technique is used, set the appropriate technical factors to be consistent with all previous phantom images.

6. Note and plot the exposure time on the chart following the exposure.

7. Process film.

8. Using the densitometer, measure the density on the film over the disk and then measure the background density, which lies adjacent to the disk. Be sure, when measuring the background density, that there are no fibrils interfering with the reading.

9. Plot the density of the background density on the control chart.

10. Plot the density difference (background density minus the density of the disk) on the control chart.

11. To score the phantom image, mask off any extraneous light from the image as if the radiologist were reading the mammogram. A magnifying lens may also be used for scoring.

12. Evaluate the film and determine how many simulated fibers, speck groups, and masses are visualized and record this on the control chart. To score the image:

    a. Count a mass as 1 point if it is identified within its correct location, its circular border is visible, and a density difference is noted.

    b. A mass is only awarded 0.5 point if it is identified within its correct location with a visible density difference, but the circular border to the mass is not visible.

    c. Count the number of objects from the largest to the smallest.

    d. Each fiber is assigned 1 point if the entire fiber length is identified in the correct location.

    e. If only one-half of the fiber is visible but the fiber is identified in its correct location, it only receives one-half of the full credit, or 0.5 point.

    f. Speck groups consist of six individual specks. If four of the six specks are identified, the group is granted a full point of 1.

    g. If only two or three specks are identifiable within a speck group, only 0.5 point is assigned to that speck group.

13. With the magnifying lens, evaluate the image for any areas that appear nonuniform and look for the presence of dirt or dust artifacts, grid lines, or any other artifacts, to perform a comparative analysis between the original and previous phantom images. Indicate any of these artifacts by circling them on the film and subtracting one from the final total for each interfering artifact.

14. If artifacts are identifiable, investigate the artifact-causing source.

ANALYSIS

For a true analysis of the phantom images, it is important that consistency is maintained. This evaluative test should always be performed and viewed by the same person with similar and consistent external factors regarding the viewing conditions/factors and also time of day the phantom is evaluated. For this test, it is important that one delegated person evaluates, scores, and charts the phantom images. However, other members within the department should also be asked to score the images on a routine basis if not a monthly basis. If a discrepancy in scores continues to occur with the other evaluators from month to month or if there is a downward trend occurring in the scoring, the Quality Control (QC) technologist should take a look at what may be the cause of this downward trend. This is when it is extremely helpful to rely on the original phantom image and the previous phantom image to do an effective comparative analysis.

Several factors to evaluate for an acceptable outcome:

1. Film density should be greater than 1.2, with control limits of ±0.20.

2. Density difference should be about 0.40, with control limits of ±0.05 allowed for a 4-mm-thick disk.

3. Each phantom image must be scored and add up to a minimum of 10 points for the outcome to be within acceptable ACR limits. ACR standards require that four fibers, three speck groups, and three masses must be identifiable, equaling a minimum final total of 10.

4. For evaluation of the simulated test objects within the phantom, the results should not decrease by more than one-half, assuming the same delegated QC technologist is performing and viewing the phantom images.

Other possible future problematic factors:

1. Any noted visual changes occurring between the current phantom image and the original film must be investigated.

2. If the density and the density difference readings exceed the suggested limits listed above, investigation of the processor, film batch, and the generator should occur and corrective action taken, if necessary.

3. If a continuous problem of visualization of grid lines, grid artifacts, artifacts, or the number of visualized simulated objects within the phantom is occurring, report this to the medical physicist for correction.

ACR requires that all phantom images be retained within the QC records for a full year.

Processor Quality Control

Processing plays an important role in film archival quality and the production of film contrast and density. It is valuable to know that the dedicated processor for mammography films is functioning to the level of the manufacturer's specifications and that the processor's function is consistent. This daily quality control test requires the use of two separate pieces of equipment, a densitometer and a sensitometer. The densitometer is used to obtain readings of densities from specific areas on a film. By plotting the required density readings, changes can be noted in contrast and speed. The sensitometer is used in the darkroom and exposes a scale of gray on a film, which gradually increases in density. The scale of gray exposed on a film is similar to the scale of gray created by a step wedge.

For an accurate assessment of a processor's functioning, a quality control strip must be performed on a daily basis. Measurable outcomes and consistency play a significant role. Quality control strips should be run each day before the arrival of patients or at least before any clinical mammograms are performed and processed. Evaluating the processor before it is in complete operation for the day allows for corrective action to be taken if necessary.

PURPOSE

To ensure that the processor is functioning to its specified maintainable limits and that the processor is consistent in its outcomes.

MATERIALS

Digital thermometer
Control box of mammographic film

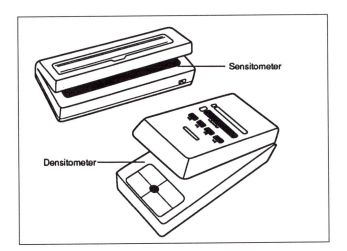

FIGURE 4-6

Sensitometer (for mammography purposes, the sensitometer should produce 21 steps in optical density in steps of 0.15)

Densitometer

Control chart

PROCEDURE

1. Check the developer temperature with a digital thermometer. Do not use a glass thermometer because the glass may break and the mercury may escape into the processor. The temperature must not differ by more than ±0.5°C from the manufacturer's specifications. Note the temperature on the control chart.

2. With a piece of film from the designated control box, place the edge of the film into the sensitometer with the emulsion side placed down or closest to the light source.

3. Process the film immediately, with the emulsion side face down and with the least exposed end of the strip fed through the processor first.

4. Be sure that the film is fed through the processor feed tray on the same side each day.

FIGURE 4-7

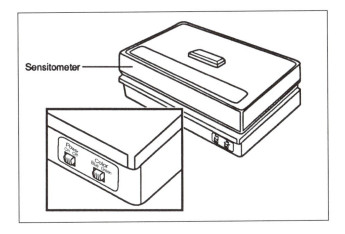

Sensitometer

FIGURE 4-8

5. Using the densitometer, measure the following three areas and record the measurements on the control chart. Remember, when measuring the steps on the sensitometric strip, always measure in the center of the step.

a. Determine which sensitometric step has a density closest to 1.20. This step will be indicated as the medium density (MD). Medium density is the speed indicator.

b. Determine which sensitometric step has a density closest to 2.20

c. Determine which sensitometric step has a density closest to, but not less than 0.45.

d. Calculate the density difference (DD) by subtracting the result from step c or the density closest to but not less than 0.45 from step b or the density step closest to 2.20. Density difference is the contrast indicator.

e. Take a density reading on any area of the film that has not been exposed by the sensitometer to obtain a base plus fog reading (B+F).

6. Record the MD, DD, and the B+F on the control chart.

If a QA program has not been established for the mammography department, the delegated QC technologist must complete the initial start-up step. Before processor quality control begins, control numbers for the control chart must be achieved. This is accomplished by first designating a control box of film. Next, for the following 5 consecutive days, a sensitometric step must be run daily. From the daily sensitometric step, figure the MD, DD, and the B+F. After the 5 days are complete, take the average of the MD, DD, and the B+F and chart these as your base control numbers.

ANALYSIS

If the plotted MD and DD fall within ±0.10 of its control limit and the B+F density is within ±0.03 of its control limit, the processor is functioning properly within its limits. However, if the MD and DD fall outside of the ±0.10 control limit but are contained within the ±0.15 limit, the test should be immediately repeated and the processor should be reevaluated due to the possibility of human error. Furthermore, if MD and DD fall outside of the ±0.15 control limit, the problem must be identified and corrected before processor can be used for clinical use. As for B+F, if the outcomes exceed the ±0.03 control limit, corrective action must be taken immediately. On the control chart, any density readings that fall outside the control limits should be indicated by circling the plotted mark on the graph and noting the possible cause of the problem in the designated area on the chart. When and if corrective action is taken, the test must be repeated and graphed to ensure that the result is now within the control limits. Be observant to any variations that may occur from day to day. If variations begin to illustrate a trend, whether it is upward or downward, the source of the problem needs to be corrected.

Processor QC charts must be kept for a complete year, and the sensitometric films for the entire month prior must be retained.

Repeat Analysis

Reject analysis must be performed in every mammography department for the purpose of tracking and identifying any consistent problems that may occur with either positioning errors or equipment failure. Through this analysis, certain factors can be improved, thus improving department efficiency and reducing patient exposure. For a proper repeat analysis, all films that required an additional image and additional radiation dose to the patient must be included in the evaluation. A repeat analysis applies to all films, not just the films rejected by the radiologists.

A repeat analysis must begin any initial QC/QA program start-up. Thereafter, a repeat analysis data should be evaluated quarterly and recorded on the QC data sheet. To obtain a valid analysis, the mammography department should have a patient quantity of at least 250 during each quarter.

PURPOSE

To collect and evaluate data to identify any consistent problems that occur from mammographic positioning or equipment and determine the means for rejection.

MATERIALS

All rejected mammography films
QC data sheet

PROCEDURE

1. Gather the collection of films for the quarterly period needed for evaluation.
2. Calculate and determine the total number of films used during the quarterly period.
3. Calculate the total number of repeat films.
4. Calculate the total number of films exposed.
5. Sort the collection of films into categories by cause: technique, positioning, artifacts, processing, good films that appear acceptable, etc.
6. From each of these categories, calculate a total for each and record.

ANALYSIS

To calculate total number of repeat rates:

$$\text{Overall repeat rate} = \frac{\text{total number of rejected films}}{\text{total number of films exposed}}$$

To calculate the percentages of repeats in each category:

$$\% \text{ repeats/category} = \frac{\text{total repeats/category}}{\text{total repeats for all categories}}$$

Repeat rates based on a 250-patient volume indicate that the overall repeat rate should be less than 2%. Category repeats rates should not exceed 5%.

Screen Cleanliness

The quality of the mammogram is quickly degraded by the appearance of artifacts within the image. Artifacts such as dirt or dust have a tendency to mimic a microcalcification within the breast tissue. Through screen cleaning, mimicking artifacts can be reduced to a minimum, resulting in the avoidance of a repeat film to determine whether the calcification is in fact a calcification or dirt or dust artifact.

Screens should be cleaned on a weekly basis or whenever screens are suspected of containing possible artifacts.

PURPOSE

To eliminate any artifact from a mammography screen that may mimic a possible pathology within the breast.

MATERIALS

Appropriate screen cleaning solution

Lint-free gauze pad or camel's hair brush

PROCEDURE

1. Remove film from screens and clean the insides of the screen. Be careful not to damage the screen by pressing too hard.

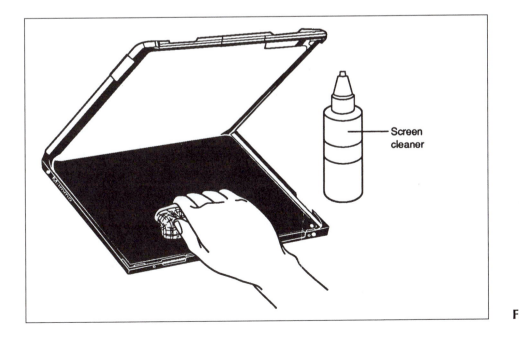

Screen cleaner

FIGURE 4-9

2. After cleaning the screen, set the cassette up vertically and only slightly opened to allow the screen to dry before closing it.

3. Once the screen is dry, load the cassette with film and allow the cassette to set for at least 15 min to allow any entrapped air to escape before use.

ANALYSIS

After screen cleaning, evaluate its effectiveness through evaluating mammographic images. Technologists should evaluate the cause of microcalcifications and determine whether it is due to artifact or pathology. Screens should be numbered individually, so evaluate the microcalcification and its location on each film.

View Box Uniformity

View boxes must be evaluated to ensure that viewing conditions are nothing less than optimum. One must maintain view boxes by evaluating consistency between all the view boxes used within a mammography department. If the amount of illumination from the technologist's view box differs from that of the radiologist, image quality may not be optimum between the two viewing stations. This results in affecting the outcome of the mammographic diagnosis.

View boxes are evaluated by the amount of illumination they provide and optimum density and contrast ranges on films. In addition to illumination, view boxes are evaluated for the overall cleanliness of the cover panel, light intensity, and the temperature of the color. The fronts of the view boxes must be cleaned to be free of any marks. The temperature of the color should be chosen to whatever hue is the most pleasing to the eye. All illuminators in each view box in each mammography department should be of the same brand and type to ensure consistent viewing conditions throughout. All illuminators should all be replaced every 2 years. All fluorescent bulbs should be replaced at the same time to ensure uniformity throughout. The intensity of the illuminators needs to maintained. If an illuminator becomes dull, visibility of detail is reduced due to increased density appearance.

Contrast is important for the diagnosis of mammographic images. To improve contrast, extraneous light must be minimized so that it does not degrade the image quality. View boxes should be positioned in areas away from windows, sources of bright light, and other view boxes.

Analysis of view box conditions should be carried out weekly.

PURPOSE

To ensure that all viewing conditions are optimum and consistent throughout to prevent a misdiagnosis because of viewing conditions.

MATERIALS

Window cleaner

Soft towel

PROCEDURE

1. Clean all view box surfaces until all marks are removed from the panel.
2. Inspect all view boxes visually for light uniformity.
3. Check and be sure that any sources of extraneous light are not reflecting off the view box fronts.

ANALYSIS

Evaluate the view boxes for uniformity and replace all bulbs at one time if dimming or flickering begins to occur within any of the bulbs. Ambient light and illuminator light can be measured with light meters. Ambient light refers to all the surrounding light conditions. Luminance is the measurement of light intensity emitted from a view box. The illuminator light reading for mammography view boxes should register to be at least 3500 nit, which will be higher than the luminance reading for diagnostic radiography. View boxes in use for diagnostic radiography will have a luminance reading of 1500 nit.

Visual Checklist

On a monthly basis, mammographic technologists need to perform a visual checklist of the department's equipment. Technologists should be certain that all the buttons, peddles, displays, and lights are working properly, consistently, and are mechanically stable.

A visual checklist of the equipment must be performed monthly and after any equipment maintenance service on mammography units.

PURPOSE

To ensure that all aspects of the mammography unit is functioning properly to maintain the patient's safety and to provide high-quality diagnostic films.

MATERIALS

Visual checklist according to the ACR manual

PROCEDURE

1. Grade the equipment by assigning a pass or fail check on the department's visual checklist after checking the functions on the C-arm, cassette holder, and the control booth.

2. For the C-arm portion of the checklist, check the SID indicator, check whether the C-arm angle is at the correct register, check whether the locks work, check whether the field light works, and check whether the C-arm moves with ease.

3. For the cassette holder portion of the checklist, check the cassette locks, grids, compression device, compression scale, and the amount of compression delivered through manual and automatic modes.

4. For the control booth portion of the checklist, check the window, panel switches, lights and meters, and the technique charts.

5. Make sure that the mammography room is supplied with means of gonadal shielding, cones, and cleaning solutions.

ANALYSIS

Each item listed on the department's visual checklist must receive a passing grade. Items on the checklist that fail to meet the passing criteria need to be immediately replaced or serviced for correction.

PART 2

Quality Management

Chapter 5   Equipment Evaluation
Chapter 6   Mammography Quality Control Procedures
Chapter 7   Artifact Assessment
Chapter 8   Processor Quality Control
Chapter 9   Statistical Analysis
Chapter 10   Federal Regulations

INTRODUCTION

Total quality management (TQM) organizations are currently incorporating total quality improvement techniques into their systems to monitor levels of quality and make continuous improvements to services or products that are produced for customers. TQM may sound as though it would apply only to the manufacturing scenes, when in fact it recently has become an integral element of the health care scene.

The term *quality* is a difficult term to define because quality is perceived differently at different levels within the marketing chain. Quality could be defined as "the totality of features and characteristics of a product/service that bear on its ability to satisfy given needs" or simply "conformance to requirements." The element of quality has always seemed to impact industries, starting back a million years.

Through the evolution of quality, early man happily accepted variation as a way of life. At this time, the human race survived in the environment by making tools and weapons out of stone. As the human race continued to evolve, individuals began making new products such as pottery, jewelry, toys, clothes, and shoes and used these products as sources of trade. Moving on to the Egyptian times, we can note that the Egyptians were one of the first civilizations to use measurement tools and systems for construction of their pyramids and other buildings. This civilization was the first to be recognized for reducing and eliminating variation in their end products because of the use of measurement tools. During the Middle Ages, those who were skilled craftsmen served as both the manufacturer and the inspector of their own products. The craftsmen were aware that their reputation, success, and income were greatly influenced by the quality of products they produced. Quality assurance at this time was very informal because each craftsman took great pride in his products and was sure to build a high level of quality into the final product.

By the 1900s, Frederick Taylor, a man who is often referred to as the "Father of Scientific Management," brought forth his philosophy on production. Taylor chose to separate the planning function from the execution stage and delegate numerous individuals to different functions or tasks within the production process. Due to the increased number of individuals involved in the process, quality assurance took a turn and largely fell into the hands of product inspectors. Inspection became the primary means of quality control during the first half of the 20th century.

After World War II, during the late 1940s and early 1950s, there was a shortage of civilian goods in the United States. This shortage of goods caused industries to focus on making production a top priority. Unfortunately, this time of mass production did not incorporate any concerns for quality or ideas of quality improvement into product manufacturing. In return, companies relied heavily on mass inspection of products.

During this same period, two quality gurus from the United States, Edward Deming and Joseph Juran, were recognized for their concepts on quality improvement efforts and quality control issues. At this time, the United States failed to recognize the importance of these concepts, but the Japanese did not. With the help of Deming and Juran, Japan began integrating quality throughout their organization and developed a culture that focused on continuous improvement efforts. The improvements the Japanese made were gradual but steady and took approximately 20 years until the results were noticeable. By 1970, due to the higher production of quality goods, the Japanese products significantly penetrated Western markets.

During the 1980s came the arrival of the United States quality revolution. This decade brought about a growing awareness of quality by U.S. consumers, industries, and the government. This awareness was due to the increase in global competition from the 1970s. When U.S. industries became aware that U.S. consumers were considering the quality of the products they were purchasing from the U.S. versus those from Japan, the government decided to turn to Deming for his assistance in running quality improvement campaigns nationwide.

From the late 1980s and through the 1990s, interest in quality has grown at an unprecedented rate. This new concern for quality and quality improvement techniques has impacted all industries, including health care.

The concepts of TQM are focused on the company-wide efforts used by companies that are concerned about achieving customer satisfaction. In 1991, JCAHO actually began incorporating the concepts of continuous quality improvement (CQI) or TQM into health care organizations. The CQI/TQM concepts are based on the "14 Points for Management" formulated by Edward Deming. The intention of incorporating CQI/TQM concepts was not intended to replace concepts of quality assurance but to incorporate the company-wide efforts of TQM on a higher level. Quality assurance and quality control efforts still play integral roles in TQM programs.

Quality assurance is a management program that strives to achieve health care excellence through the collection and evaluation of data. Its primary focus is the deliverance of quality of care to customers even though it directly relies on parameters involving health care employees. Quality assurance programs, similar to TQM programs, focus on reducing or eliminating any variations that occur within a process or system due to human efforts.

Quality control is a subcomponent of quality assurance programs and deals specifically with any technical elements and the maintenance of these technical elements, i.e., instruments and equipment.

Total quality management focuses on the needs and expectations of the customer for continuous improvement efforts made toward products or services. TQM organizations focus on making continual adjustments to products or services according to the voice of the customer obtained through survey or questionnaire analysis. Organizations that have adopted TQM principles have been able to reduce operating expenses for the organization and improve customer satisfaction. TQM is a structured and systematic approach in which all employees are consulted and empowered for sources of ideas to continually aid in the needed improvement processes.

A portion of TQM focuses on the formulation of new processes within our departments to improve final outcomes such as customer satisfaction and the deliverance of high-quality care. A *process* is a sequential series of steps that must take place to achieve a desired outcome. Any process involves a supplier, input, action, output, and the customer. A *supplier* may be a company or individual who provides the institution with goods or services. The *input* portion of the process provides any information that may be pertinent for reaching the final outcome. *Action* is simply the means that activity organizations go through to reach the final outcome. The *output* is the final outcome or product obtained from completing the three previous steps. Finally, there is always a *customer* inherent within a process. Customers can be either internal or external to the facility. Internal and external customers will be covered later in the text.

Through TQM efforts, organizations empower employees to contribute knowledge toward existing processes and formulate new ideas for better replacement processes. Some TQM organizations may take part in the concept of benchmarking. *Benchmarking* allows organizations to measure their performance standards against those that are within their competitive market. Organizations may even choose to adopt ready-made processes that are successful from other organizations and implement them into their own processes.

TQM is concept that requires company-wide involvement, beginning with the understanding of TQM principles by top management. TQM management styles have replaced traditional management techniques by eliminating the bureaucratic steps of management. TQM managers must act as facilitators rather than leaders of the organization. TQM managers must also empower employees to improve the overall success of the organization. Employee empowerment will not only benefit the institution, it will also create motivation, improve job satisfaction, and improve the overall employee morale, thereby enabling all to work better as a team rather than as individuals.

CHAPTER 5
Equipment Evaluation

Automatic Exposure Control

Automatic exposure control (AEC) allows the amount of radiation that penetrates the patient to be measured as current. A required, precalibrated amount of current will determine specific densities produced on a film. When the current charges a capacitor to the predetermined level, an electronic switch terminates the exposure.

AEC should be established when the equipment is installed and evaluated semiannually to ensure minimal patient exposure. The tests most commonly used to evaluate AEC include but are not limited to back-up exposure time, minimum exposure time, and exposure consistency.

PURPOSE

The purpose of evaluating the AEC is to ensure that consistent radiographic density levels and minimum exposure levels are maintained.

Consistency of Chambers

MATERIALS

Energized radiographic unit

One 10 × 12 radiographic cassette

Processor

Phantom (large enough to cover a single ionization chamber)

Densitometer

PROCEDURE

1. To evaluate the consistency of the chambers, three exposures should be made, using each chamber separately.
2. The phantom should be placed over the chamber being evaluated.

3. The film should be in the bucky and a 40 in. source-to-image distance (SID) should be established.

4. Technical factors and density settings should be consistent for each exposure.

5. The same cassette should be used for each exposure to minimize the effect of outside variables.

6. The three exposures should be evaluated with a densitometer. Optical density should not differ by more than ±20%.

Consistency of Exposure
with Variable Anatomical Thickness

MATERIALS

Energized radiographic unit
One 10 × 12 radiographic cassette
Processor
Phantoms of different thicknesses
Densitometer

PROCEDURE

1. To evaluate the consistency of the AEC, the same chamber(s) should be used, but different part thicknesses are employed

2. The phantom should be placed over the chamber.

3. The film should be in the bucky, and a 40 in. SID should be established.

4. Technical factors and density settings should be consistent for each exposure.

5. The same cassette should be used for each exposure to minimize the effect of outside variables.

6. The three exposures should be evaluated with a densitometer. Optical density should not differ by more than ±20%.

Exposure Consistency with Variable Milliamperage

MATERIALS

Energized radiographic unit

One 11 × 14 radiographic cassette

Processor

Phantom

Densitometer

PROCEDURE

1. To evaluate the consistency of the AEC, the same chamber(s) should be used with various different milliampere stations.

2. The phantom should be placed over the chamber.

3. The film should be in the bucky, and a 40 in. SID should be established.

4. The milliampere station will differ with each exposure, but all other technical factors and density settings should remain unchanged.

5. The same cassette should be used for each exposure to minimize the effect of outside variables.

6. The three exposures should be evaluated with a densitometer. Optical density should not differ by more than ±20%.

Exposure Consistency with Variable Kilovoltage

MATERIALS

Energized radiographic unit

One 11 × 14 radiographic cassette

Processor

Phantom

Densitometer

PROCEDURE

1. To evaluate the consistency of the AEC, the same chamber(s) should be used with different kilovolt stations (70, 80, and 90 kVp).
2. The phantom should be placed over the chamber.
3. The film should be in the bucky, and a 40 in. SID should be established.
4. The kilovolt station will differ with each exposure, but all other technical factors and density settings should remain unchanged.
5. The same cassette should be used for each exposure to minimize the effect of outside variables.
6. The three exposures should be evaluated with a densitometer. Optical density should not differ by more than ±20%.

Back-Up Timer (Maximum Exposure Time)

MATERIALS

Energized radiographic unit

Stop watch

Lead apron or shield large enough to cover all chambers

PROCEDURE

1. To evaluate the back-up or maximum exposure time allowed, one should use a stopwatch to ensure that the back-up time set is actually acquired.
2. The lead should be placed over the chambers.
3. A 40 in. SID should be established.
4. An exposure using 75 kVp at 100 mA and a back-up time of 6 s should be set.
5. The three exposures should be evaluated with a densitometer.
6. The exposure should terminate at 6 s or 600 mA.

Minimum Exposure Times

The manufacturer usually specifies minimum exposure time and milliampere combinations. Time settings below 10 ms using AEC will usually fail to produce consistent densities.

Timer Evaluation

Because the timer controls the duration of radiographic exposure, it is important to evaluate it for accuracy to ensure proper density and radiation dose. *All timers should be within ±5% of what is set for times above 10 ms and ±10% for times below 10 ms.*

Single-Phase Generator Testing

SPINNING TOP

Because single-phase equipment produces a pulse of energy for each cycle of the sine wave, a dot can be produced by using the manual spinning top. The type of rectification, waveform, and length of time used determines the number of dots.

MATERIALS

Energized radiographic unit

Manual spinning top

10 × 12 cassette

PROCEDURE

1. The loaded cassette should be placed atop the table, and a 40 in. SID employed.

2. The spinning top is placed on the cassette within the field light.

3. The top should be spun at a rate that will allow it to keep spinning throughout the exposure.

4. Two exposures can be made on the cassette providing proper collimation is used.

5. To minimize outside variables, one cassette should be used, which will require the evaluator to run the film after the first two exposures are made.

6. Exposures should be made using the same SID, kilovoltage, and milliampere station. Four exposures, one at each of the following time settings, should be made: 1/10, 1/20, 1/30, and 1/40.

7. Process the film and evaluate the number of dots recorded.

8. The following formulas should be used with the type of equipment specified:

Half-wave rectification exposure time $\times$ 60 = correct number of dots produced

Full-wave rectification exposure time $\times$ 120 = correct number of dots produced

With half-wave rectification, one useful pulse is recorded per cycle; with full-wave rectification, two useful pulses are recorded per cycle.

Three-Phase and High-Frequency Generator Testing

Synchronous Motor-Driven Spinning Top

Three-phase and high-frequency power do not produce a pulse of energy, but a continuous amount of energy over the time that is set. For this reason, it is not possible to use the manual spinning top to test this type of equipment. A synchronous top is used. This electrical tool rotates at a constant rate of speed (1 revolution/s) throughout the time that is set. An arch or series of slits will appear on the test radiograph.

MATERIALS

Energized radiographic unit

Synchronous motor-driven tool

Extension cord

10 × 12 cassette

PROCEDURE

1. The loaded cassette should be placed atop the table and a 40 in. SID employed.
2. The synchronous top is placed on the cassette within the field light.
3. Two exposures can be made on the cassette providing proper collimation is used.
4. To minimize outside variables, one cassette should be used, which will require the evaluator to run the film after the first two exposures are made.
5. Exposures should be made using the same SID, kilovoltage, and milliampere station. Four exposures, one at each of the following time settings, should be made: 1/10, 1/20, 1/30, and 1/40.
6. Process the film and evaluate film
7. The following formula should be used with three-phase type of equipment:

$$\text{size of arch recorded} = \text{exposure time} \times 360°.$$

It is important to realize that, because the synchronous disk spins at 1 revolution/s, one full arch will be recorded when using a 1 s exposure time. The length of the arch should correspond with the amount of time used. Usually a protractor or template is used to measure the recorded arch.

Digital Meter/Oscilloscope

With three-phase multipulse and high-frequency units, many evaluators will choose to use the digital milliampere meter. This tool allows for evaluation of the milliampere output when microprocessors instead of timers regulate the duration of exposure. The oscilloscope allows for display of the waveform that will verify and extensively evaluate the generator. Both tools should be used only by a qualified technologist.

Half-Value Layer

The half-value layer (HVL) is commonly defined as the amount of filtration required to reduce the intensity of the x-ray beam by one-half its original value. One should realize that the HVL is an expression of the quality or intensity of the beam. As beam quality increases, the HVL must be increased to reduce the intensity. The HVL is actually a representation of the quality of the beam.

Evaluation of the HVL is necessary to ensure that proper beam filtration is used and should be done when the equipment is installed and then annually.

MATERIALS

Graph paper

Dosimeter pencil

Aluminum filters (1.0 mm thick)

Lead apron or shield

Energized radiographic unit

PROCEDURE

1. SID should be 40 inches.
2. The dosimeter pencil should be placed directly in the radiated area.
3. A lead shield should be under the dosimeter on the tabletop to prevent higher readings attributed to scatter radiation.
4. The field should be collimated so as to include the entire dosimeter, with the light slightly greater than the dosimeter.
5. Technical factors should be set to obtain an exposure, which allows a reading of 90% on the dosimeter scale; 70 kVp and 60 mA employing a long exposure time should suffice.
6. Expose the dosimeter and record the value. Reset the dosimeter.
7. One millimeter of aluminum should be added and a subsequent exposure made.
8. The data should be recorded and a series of exposures made by adding 1 mm of aluminum each time until the data from a total of 8.0 mm of aluminum are recorded.
9. Using the graph paper, prepare a logarithmic curve evaluating the thickness of the lead or HVL (x axis) and the amount of radiation detected (y axis).

10. Record the exposure to the amount of lead used on the curve for each exposure taken.

11. The HVL is determined by subtracting the value of aluminum used when the amount of radiation detected was one-half of the original from the amount of aluminum used to filter the greatest amount of detected radiation.

Grid Uniformity Evaluation

For the grid to properly filter scatter photons, the lead strips must be uniform in their linearity. Warped, bent, or cracked grids may distort or obstruct pathology important to radiographic quality and diagnosis. The density readings used to evaluate the uniformity of a grid should be with ±10% of the optimal value.

MATERIALS

Energized radiographic unit

Processor

Grids to be evaluated

Cassettes to fit grid size

Densitometer

Phantom or plastic pan of water

PROCEDURE

1. Place the cassette under the grid, within the grid cap, or the grid cassette.
2. A 40 in. SID should be used, and enough technique should be used to produce an optical density of 1.0 despite the grid ratio of the grid being evaluated.
3. The phantom or pan of water should then be placed on top of the grid and an image produced.
4. After processing the image, it should be visually inspected for areas of nonuniformity that will produce an area of greater radiographic density
5. The image should then be divided into four quadrants.
6. Optical density readings of each quadrant should be produced with a densitometer.
7. All readings should fall within the specified standards.

Field Light Accuracy

Shutters within the collimator assembly control the field light. It is imperative, because the field light represents the size of the irradiated field, that accuracy of the field be inspected for both alignment and perpendicularity of the beam. Testing the alignment can be done with the nine-penny test or a collimator test tool. Perpendicularity can be evaluated most accurately with a beam alignment and collimator test tool. Field light accuracy and perpendicularity must be within 2% of the SID employed.

Field Light Alignment

The field light may be evaluated with a collimator test tool. This template has incremental measurements within it that will appear on the test radiograph after processing. Any radiopaque object can be used in place of the template. Paper clips and pennies are commonly used.

MATERIALS

Energized radiographic unit

Processor

Template or radiopaque objects

10 × 12 cassettes loaded with medium-speed film

PROCEDURE

1. The loaded cassette should be placed within the table bucky.
2. A 40 in. SID is employed, as are technical factors that allow for an optical density of 1.5 to be produced.
3. The collimators should be adjusted to an 8 × 10 field size, with the template centered in the field light, cross hairs to the middle.
4. Measure the actual field size projected from the center to each side of the film. Record the data.
5. The film should be marked to identify any misalignment.
6. If using radiopaque objects, they should be aligned with the outer margins of the field light.
7. If using pennies, place a penny on the north, south, east, and west points on the outside the collimated field. Place corresponding pennies on the same points on the inside of the collimated field. One penny should also be positioned in the middle of the field light where the cross hairs intersect.

8. Expose the radiograph. If using radiopaque objects, remove the objects and expose the film a second time with the collimators open to the actual film size before processing. (This will allow for visualization of any object that may otherwise be collimated out of the field due to misalignment of projected field.)

9. After the film has been processed, measure the irradiated field size from the center to each of the four sides of the film. Record the data.

10. Compare the actual projected field size with the irradiated field size. Any misalignment should be noted, and misrepresentation of the field size should be noted.

11. Compare the results with the allowable standards. Failure to fall within the specific standards warrants contacting a qualified service representative for correction.

Beam Perpendicularity

The perpendicularity of the beam should be evaluated to ensure that the beam is meeting the imaging device in a perpendicular plane. The metallic objects mounted in the alignment test tool should be within 0.5° of one another or within the two most inner circles of the template to be considered satisfactory.

MATERIALS

Energized radiographic unit

Processor

Template and alignment test tool (cylinder with two metallic pellets mounted in each end)

10 × 12 medium-speed cassettes loaded with film

PROCEDURE

1. The loaded cassette should be placed within the table bucky.
2. A 40 in. SID is employed, as are technical factors that will allow for an optical density of 1.5 to be produced.
3. The collimators should be adjusted to an 8 × 10 field size, with the template centered in the field light, cross hairs to the middle.
4. The collimator test tool should be placed on top and in the center of the template.
5. The film should be marked to identify any misalignment.
6. After the film has been processed, evaluate the alignment of the metallic pellets. They should fall directly on top or within close proximity to one another within the circles of the template. Record the data.
7. Compare the results with the allowable standards. Failure to fall within the specific standards warrants contacting a qualified service representative for correction.

Milliampere Linearity Evaluation

PURPOSE

The purpose of this specific milliamperage check is to evaluate the linearity of milliampere stations by altering the station but keeping all other variables constant. Because the relation between milliampere and density is proportional, if all other variables are constant and the milliampere station is changed, one should be able to evaluate efficiency based on density readings. Results must be within ±10% of the standard.

MATERIALS

Energized radiographic unit

Processor

10 × 12 medium-speed cassette and film

Penetrometer

Densitometer

PROCEDURE

1. Three exposures are made on the film. Lead strips should be used to shield portions not being irradiated.
2. The film should be placed on the tabletop and divided into three equal portions with the lead strips.
3. Prepare the first one-third of the cassette to be exposed by placing the penetrometer in the center of the area being exposed.
4. Technical factors should allow for a median optical density of 1.5 at a distance of 40 inches. The only factor that should be changed is the milliampere station.
5. The first exposure should use a 50 mA station. The second and third exposures will use a 100 and 200 mA station.
6. The penetrometer should be placed in the center of the irradiated portion of the cassette for each exposure. Each exposure should be marked with a lead number.
7. Process the film and read each of the penetrometer steps between 0.7 and 2.5 for each of the three exposures.
8. Record the steps of each of the three test images taken.
9. Using the second test image as a standard, compare these data with those from the other two. The percentage differences should fall within the specified range.
10. An optical density increase of 0.3 equals doubling the radiographic density. An optical density decrease of 0.3 equals halving the radiographic density.

Milliamperage and Seconds Reciprocity

PURPOSE

The law of reciprocity states that different milliampere and time combinations will produce the same milliamperage and therefore should produce the same density. When evaluating milliamperage reciprocity, different milliampere and time stations are used to produce the same milliamperes. A densitometer and penetrometer are used to evaluate the radiographic densities produced. Densities should be within ±10% of one another.

MATERIALS

Energized radiographic unit

Processor

Densitometer

Penetrometer

10 × 12 cardboard cassette

PROCEDURE

1. Three exposures are made on the film. Lead strips should be used to shield portions not being irradiated.
2. The film should be placed on the tabletop and divided into three equal portions with the lead strips.
3. Prepare the first one-third of the cassette to be exposed by placing the penetrometer in the center of the area being exposed.
4. Technical factors should allow for a median optical density of 1.5 at a distance of 55 inches.
5. All exposures should be produced with the same kilovoltage and 50 mA.
6. The penetrometer should be placed in the center of the irradiated portion of the cassette for each exposure. Each exposure should be marked with a lead number.
7. Process the film.
8. Record the optical density of steps at densities of 0.8–2.0 on each of the three test images taken. An average of these steps for each of the three test exposures should be calculated. This will be the mean.

CHAPTER 5   EQUIPMENT EVALUATION

9. Using the midrange density as a standard, determine the percentage difference by subtracting the optical density of the step with the minimum density from the optical density of the step with the maximum density. Divide this number by 2 and then divide by the mean. To find the percentage, one should multiply the difference by 100.

10. An optical density increase of 0.3 equals doubling the radiographic density. An optical density decrease of 0.3 equals halving the radiographic density.

Milliampere Reproducibility

Evaluating milliampere reproducibility involves consistency of output using the same milliamperage and time station and to make a series of exposures. The output should not differ by more than ±5%.

MATERIALS

Energized radiographic unit

Processor

Densitometer

Penetrometer

10×12 medium-speed cassette and film

PROCEDURE

1. Three exposures are made on the film. Lead strips should be used to shield portions not being irradiated.

2. The film should be placed on the tabletop and divided into three equal portions with the lead strips.

3. Prepare the first one-third of the cassette to be exposed by placing the penetrometer in the center of the area being exposed.

4. Technical factors should allow for a median optical density of 1.5 at a distance of 40 inches.

5. The penetrometer should be placed in the center of the irradiated portion of the cassette for each exposure. Each exposure should be marked with a lead number.

6. All exposures should be produced with the same kilovoltage and milliamperage.

7. Process the film.

8. Record the optical density of steps with densities of 0.8–2.0 on each of the three test images taken. An average of these steps for each of the three test exposures should be calculated.

9. These averages should not deviate by more than ±5%.

Kilovoltage Accuracy Evaluation

Three instruments can be used to noninvasively evaluate the accuracy of kilovoltage output. These are the penetrometer, the wide-range cassette (Adran and Crooke's or Wisconsin), and the digital kilovoltage meter. It is important that the kilovoltage set is consistent with that produced. Kilovoltage is the primary factor that controls image contrast, and it has an effect on patient dose because of the influence kilovoltage has on beam penetration and image density. Variations between the kilovoltage set and that produced should be ±5%.

Evaluation with the Penetrometer

PROCEDURE

Although the penetrometer is the simplest test, it is also the least accurate. The kilovoltage produced may differ from that which is set. This test evaluates the ability of the unit to produce consistent density and contrast at a given kilovoltage setting when using different milliampere and time values while maintaining milliamperage. Because this method is not an accurate way to assess kilovoltage, the only procedures explained in this section will be the wide-range cassette and the digital kilovoltage meter.

Evaluation with the Wisconsin Cassette

The Wisconsin cassette is specially designed to attenuate the light produced by the screens as they interact with the photon energies of the beam. Most wide-range cassettes can test a range of kilovolt settings. The beam is attenuated at different rates by different thicknesses of copper depending on the level of kilovoltage being evaluated. The basic concept is that one can assess beam penetrability by assessing the amount of attenuation by the copper step wedges versus optical attenuation. A series of densities is produced from each method of attenuation. A comparison is made between the two series of densities (dots) produced.

MATERIALS

Energized radiographic unit
Processor
Wisconsin (wide-range) cassette
Densitometer
Lead shields
Film for cassette

PROCEDURE

1. If a wide-range cassette is used, a 40 in. SID is employed. The milliamperage should produce a density of 1.0 in the reference column of the cassette. The kilovoltage should be appropriate for the level being evaluated. A 20 in. SID should be used for fixed kilovoltage assessment tools.

2. Load the cassette with medium-speed film and place the cassette on the tabletop so that the anode and cathode run along the long axis of the cassette.

3. All portions of the cassette should be masked accept for the 60 kVp section. Expose this section using 60 kVp.

4. Expose the next section, after covering all other portions, by using the appropriate amount of kilovoltage and a milliampere that will produce and an optical density close to 1.0.

5. Expose the remaining sections as indicated in the previous step, ensuring that all areas except the test area are covered. Make sure the kilovoltage is adjusted according to the level being evaluated.

6. Process the radiograph.

7. Using the densitometer, record the density of the dots in the test column and in the reference column. Find the set of dots that corresponds most in value. It may be necessary to find the average of the densities in the reference column, if they differ slightly.

8. Determine the step at which both densities best correspond for each test area. Record this level.

9. Using the interpretation instrument or graph provided, plot and interpret the results.

Evaluation with a Digital Kilovoltage Meter

The digital kilovoltage meter displays the kilovoltage output and has the ability to demonstrate whether the kilovoltage set is within the range of that produced. The kilovoltage output is digitally displayed on the face of the meter. The meter is the easiest of all kilovoltage measuring instruments to use and has a high degree of accuracy. Radiographic film and means of processing are not required.

MATERIALS

Digital kilovoltage meter

Energized radiographic unit

PROCEDURE

1. Place the digital meter on the tabletop directly under the x-ray beam.

2. Center the beam to the cross hairs on the top of the meter.

3. Select the appropriate kilovoltage to be evaluated.

4. Select the type of generator power being used and depress the corresponding button on the face of the meter.

5. Warm up the meter with an exposure of at least 100 mA and 100 kVp.

6. When testing the kilovoltage, expose the meter to a minimum exposure time of 0.02 s.

7. Set the desired technical factors and expose the meter.

8. The actual kilovoltage produced will be displayed on the face of the meter.

9. Compare the kilovoltage produced with the kilovoltage set and verify that specifications are met.

View Box Uniformity Evaluation

The view box should be cleaned and evaluated annually. All bulbs should be replaced every 2 years. The luminance of each view box within the department must not differ by more than ±15%. The luminance within the four quadrants of a single view box should not differ by more than ±10%. Within banks of view boxes, the luminance should not differ by more than ±20%.

View box luminance for radiography should be at a minimum of 1500 nit, and luminance for mammography view boxes should be no less than 3500 nit.

View box illuminance should be at least 5000 lx, or 500 ft-cd.

The ambient light levels within a viewing area should be 320 lx (or 30 ft-cd) and mammography should be 50 lx.

Terms

Lumen	unit of luminous flux measured in candles or candelas
Illuminance	amount of flux per unit of area on a given surface, measured in lux (lumens/m^2) or foot-candles (ft-cd)
Luminance	intensity per unit of area on a given surface, measure in candles/cm^2 or nit

MATERIALS

Photometer (photo light meter)

View boxes

Electrical outlet

Cardboard mask (14 × 17 piece of cardboard divided into four quadrants with a small hole in the center of each quadrant)

PROCEDURE

1. All view boxes should be disassembled and cleaned before measuring luminance.
2. The cardboard mask should be placed over the view box to be evaluated.
3. Place the light meter over the hole in each quadrant of the mask and record the level of luminescence for each quadrant.

4. Repeat this procedure for each view box being evaluated and record the results.

5. To determine the average luminescence for a single view box, add each of the four results recorded for each quadrant and divide by four.

6. To determine the results for a bank of view boxes, find the average luminescence for each of the view boxes in the bank and divide by the total number of view boxes in the bank.

CHAPTER 6

Mammography Quality Control Procedures

Compression

Compression is used to reduce the thickness of the breast tissue, which is essential for the production of a high-quality mammogram. Through compression tissue thickness is decreased, resulting in decreased patient dose and increased image contrast, quality, and sharpness. At present, all mammography units must be equipped with a compression device that allows mammographers to apply gentle pressure to the breast to obtain quality mammograms. However, because compression is applied for many examinations, it is essential to maintain image quality. Mammographers can ensure that adequate compression is maintained through testing both the manual adjustments and the powered mode. Most importantly, one can ensure that the equipment does not allow too much compression to be applied.

This test should be performed initially with any new equipment, semiannually, and when reduced compression is suspected.

PURPOSE

To evaluate and ensure that adequate compression is maintained through testing both the manual adjustment and the powered mode. Whether compression is checked through the powered mode or manual mode, the compression should meet a minimum of 25 lbs. and a maximum of 40 lbs. Most importantly, ensure that the equipment does not allow too much compression to be applied.

MATERIALS

Flat bathroom scale
Towels
Mammography unit

PROCEDURE

1. Place a towel on the cassette holder to protect it.
2. Place the bathroom scale on the towel with the dial facing out for easy reading and make sure that the center of the scale is located directly under the compression device.
3. Place one or more towels on top of the scale to protect the compression device.
4. Using the power drive, allow the compression device to compress until it stops automatically.
5. Read and record the compression in pounds and then release the compression.
6. Using the manual drive, move the compression device down until it cannot compress any more.
7. Read and record the compression in pounds and then release the compression.

ANALYSIS

To evaluate adequate compression in the power drive mode, the compression should range anywhere from 25 to 40 lbs. to be within acceptable limits. To evaluate the compression under manual drive, compression of at least 25 lbs. should be achievable, and compressions up to 40 lbs. are acceptable.

If the test fails to meet these criteria, a service engineer should be contacted to make the appropriate internal adjustments.

Darkroom Cleanliness

Minimizing artifacts that mimic microcalcifications begins with and depends on darkroom cleanliness. Mammographic images reflect how well the darkroom is maintained. Darkrooms must be maintained by daily cleaning of the countertops, processor feed trays, pass boxes, floors, and a weekly cleaning of air vents and safelights. Construction of the darkroom is also an important factor that must be kept in mind. It is important that neither heating nor air-conditioning vents are installed above the countertops or the processor feed trays. Ceilings should be constructed of a solid material to reduce any dust or other particles from falling on work surfaces. Storage space or cabinets should not be installed above the countertops. These storage spaces create a place where dust may accumulate.

This test should be performed daily each workday before patients are seen.

PURPOSE

To minimize artifacts on an image that may cause misdiagnosis.

MATERIALS

Wet mop and pail

Lint-free towels

PROCEDURE

1. Damp mop the floor (daily) and walls (weekly) if dust is a problem.
2. Remove all items from the countertop and work areas.
3. With a clean, damp towel wipe off countertops and processor feed trays and wipe out the inside of the pass boxes. *Make sure that your hands remain clean.*
4. Once a week, either wipe off or vacuum the overhead air vents and safelights. Remember to do this before proceeding with the daily routine cleaning of the darkroom.

ANALYSIS

Darkroom cleanliness is evaluated best through screen cleanliness. Evaluate films for dust and dirt artifacts that appear on mammographic images.

Darkroom Fog

Every darkroom should be inspected for darkroom fog on a regular basis to ensure that outside light sources or the safelighting within the room are not fogging the mammographic film. During this inspection, it is important to evaluate all safelights to ensure that they are mounted at the appropriate distance from the workspace. Also, ensure that the safelight filters are not cracked. Cracked safelights or other sources of white-light leaks result in the fogging of film, which decreases the contrast of a piece of film, which creates differences in densities between one film and the next. Different sheets of film may demonstrate more or less density depending on the amount of fog exposure.

This test should be performed initially and semiannually thereafter. This test should also be performed when safelight bulbs or filters are changed or whenever fog may be suspected.

PURPOSE

The purpose is to evaluate and ensure that the mammographic film is not exposed to any fogging light sources inside or outside the darkroom.

MATERIALS

Densitometer

Mammographic film (from an unopened box)

Opaque card

Watch

PROCEDURE

1. Be sure that the safelight bulb wattage is correct and that the filters do not appear cracked or faded.
2. Check for the correct distance between the safelight and the countertops.
3. Turn off all the lights in the darkroom. Before beginning, allow 5 min to pass so the eyes can adjust.
4. Inspect the darkroom for any obvious light leaks that may be occurring. Check around the doors, pass boxes, processors, and the ceiling. When checking for light leaks, evaluate for leaks from different aspects of the room to ensure that it has been inspected thoroughly.
5. Fix any and all light leaks before proceeding with the test.
6. Check for any afterglow that may be occurring with the darkroom's overhead fluorescent lights by turning the lights on for 2 min and then turning them off.

7. Load a cassette with the appropriate film in total darkness.

8. Exit the darkroom and make an exposure using the phantom. Place the phantom on the cassette holder and make sure that the phantom is lined up evenly with the chest wall side of the cassette.

9. Bring compression down atop the phantom.

10. Either set the manual exposure time and milliamperage or place the phototimer sensor in the appropriate position to match all previously run tests for a 4–4.5 cm compressed breast. Consistency is very important.

11. Return to the darkroom and remove the exposed film and lay it on the counter with the emulsion side facing up. Cover one-half of the phantom image with the opaque card so that the card is perpendicular to the chest wall edge of the film.

12. With the safelights on, allow the film to lay on the countertop for 2 min.

13. Process the film.

14. After the film is processed, use the densitometer to measure close to the dividing edge, which separates the fogged from the unfogged portion of the phantom. When measuring with the densitometer, try not to measure close to any test objects within the phantom.

15. In a similar manner, also measure the density of the fogged portion to the unfogged portion. When obtaining this measurement, be sure to place the densitometer at a spot adjacent to the boundary of the opaque card.

16. Determine the amount of fog by subtracting the density of the unfogged portion from the fogged portion of the phantom.

ANALYSIS

The density difference obtained from the last step of the procedure should not be greater than 0.05. If the density difference is greater than 0.05, there must be an evident source of fog, which must be determined and corrected. Reexamine the darkroom for any light leaks, safelight imperfections, and the correct safelight bulb wattage. This test will indicate the length of time a film may be "safe" within the darkroom conditions.

Film–Screen Contact

Mammography requires a consistent level of quality to be maintained. In any modality but especially mammography, film–screen contact must be maintained for purposes of detail and spatial resolution. Film–screen contact significantly affects the image sharpness. In mammography, film–screen systems have a higher spatial resolution of 16–20 cycles/mm as opposed to only 4–8 cycles/mm for conventional systems. However, to maintain either level of resolution, the film and the screen must remain in the closest contact with one another.

This test should be performed initially with any new cassettes. Cassettes should also be evaluated on a semiannual basis and anytime thereafter when decreased image sharpness is suspected.

PURPOSE

To ensure that all mammographic cassettes are producing the highest image quality by ensuring that proper film–screen contact is occurring.

MATERIALS

Copper screen mesh consisting of 40 wires per inch

Acrylic sheets 4 cm thick to ensure a reasonable exposure time

Densitometer

All screens and cassettes to be tested

Mammography film

PROCEDURE

1. Begin by carefully cleaning all screens and cassettes with a screen cleaner. Be sure that the insides of the cassettes are cleaned thoroughly.
2. Allow the insides of the screens to air dry for approximately 30 min before closing or loading the cassettes with film.
3. Load all the cassettes with the appropriate film size.
4. Allow the cassettes to sit for 15 min so that any air trapped within the cassettes can escape.
5. One at a time, lay the cassettes atop of the cassette holder (bucky/grid). Do not use the grid for this test.
6. Place the wire mesh directly on top of the cassette so that it is centered on the cassette.

7. Place the acrylic sheet (only if needed) on top of the compression paddle and then raise the compression paddle and position it close the tube port. The acrylic sheet is used to ensure an exposure time of at least 0.5 s and to produce an optical density of 0.70–0.80 over the area of the mesh nearest the chest wall side of the film. The acrylic sheet will also aid in minimizing the amount of scatter radiation reaching the film.

8. Select a manual technique setting that will provide optical film density of 0.70–0.80 nearest the chest wall edge of the radiograph. Use 25–28 kVp.

9. Expose and process the film.

10. Continue to repeat these first nine steps on each cassette to be tested.

11. Hang the exposed radiographs on the view box and stand back at least 3 ft to evaluate. During the evaluation, look for any areas that appear "blurry" or even dark. Either sign will indicate areas of poor film–screen contact.

ANALYSIS

Areas on the films that represent poor film–screen contact and that measure more than 1 cm in diameter should first be retested. The entire procedure should then be repeated, beginning with cleaning the screen and cassette. Once the cassette is retested and the large area of poor film–screen contact has not been eliminated, this cassette should be taken out of use and replaced. If films present five or more areas of poor film–screen contact and measure less than 1 cm in diameter, they are still within acceptable limits. Often the darkened areas that measure less than 1 cm represent poor screen cleaning and are signs of dirt or dust. Poor film–screen contact can also result from damaged cassettes, deterioration of foam within the cassette, which does not allow for sufficient equalized pressure, or air trapped within the cassette.

Fixer Retention

Fixer ingredients allow for silver halide crystals to be removed from the film. This agent affects silver recovery and replenishment rates. If fixing agents are not removed from the film in the wash cycle; a yellowing or tarnishing of the film may be evident. This yellowing is due to a chemical reaction between thiosulfate and silver in the emulsion producing silver sulfide, which is responsible for the staining of the image.

This test should be performed quarterly. The American National Standards Institute (ANSI) recommends that the acceptable limit of residual hypo be less than 2 $\mu g/cm^2$ for diagnostic radiography and 5 μ/cm^2 for mammography.

PURPOSE

The purpose of the fixer retention test is to evaluate the quantity of residual fixer in a processed film.

MATERIALS

A commercial hypo retention kit may be purchased

To make your own kit, use the following recipe; ingredients can be obtained from a photographic supply store: 75 mL distilled water, 12.5 mL 28% acetic acid, and 0.75 g silver nitrate. Combine and stir distilled water and acetic acid, add silver nitrate while stirring, and continue to stir until all is dissolved. To this solution add enough distilled water to create a total solution of 100 mL. Store in a dark container in a cool dark environment.

Hypo indicator strip (if not using kit)

8 × 10 film

Processor

PROCEDURE

1. Remove the film directly from the film bin and process.
2. After the film has been processed, place one drop of hypo test solution on the film.
3. If using single emulsion film, the solution should be placed on the emulsion side.
4. If using dual emulsion film, each side must be tested individually. Solution should be placed so that it does not interfere with the area being tested on the opposite side.
5. Allow the solution to stand for 2 min.

6. Excess solution should be removed by blotting with a cloth. Do not rub.

7. Place stained area over a white sheet of paper and lay the hypo indicator strip so that a comparative analysis can be done.

8. Analysis should be done immediately because light will cause the stain to darken.

ANALYSIS

If the test indicates that levels are not within the guidelines, repeat the test immediately. If a similar test result is obtained, corrective measures should be taken. Troubleshooting measures may include evaluating:

1. The wash tank to ensure correct water levels.
2. The wash water flow rate to ensure that it is set to the manufacturer's guidelines.
3. The fixer replenishment rate to ensure that it is set to manufacturer's guidelines.

If all appear to be correct, the processor may not be the problem. Consult the film manufacturer for possible suggestions.

Phantom Imaging

Phantom imaging is one of the most important factors of mammography quality assurance. Performance of the test allows for evaluation of resolution, contrast, density changes, uniformity, and possible tube degeneration. By using a phantom, the output of the mammography units can be evaluated over a period of time and units may be maintained.

This test should be performed initially after equipment calibration. To establish a baseline level, the processor should be filled with fresh chemistry at the time the equipment is calibrated. Once the baseline is achieved, the phantom testing should be performed at least monthly or anytime when equipment (processors or units) is serviced or when fluctuation of image quality is suspected.

Purpose

To establish a baseline of quality that allows for evaluation of the equipment involved with the entire imaging chain over a period of time to ensure that the equipment is functioning properly and to maintain the highest level of quality achievable.

Materials

Mammography-accredited phantom (a square acrylic block filled with a variety of simulated masses, fibers, and specks, which is equivalent in size to a 4–4.5 cm compressed breast)

Acrylic disk (1 cm in diameter and 4 mm thick, to create a density difference)

Mammography cassette loaded with film

Original phantom image

Previous phantom image

Densitometer

Control charts

Magnifying lens

Procedure

1. Position the loaded cassette in the cassette holder of the bucky.
2. Secure the 4 mm thick acrylic disk on the phantom consistent with its placement on all previous phantom films taken. It is important to place the acrylic disk in an area on the phantom that does not interfere with any of details of the phantom. *Suggestion: Secure the acrylic disk to the phantom with glue so consistent location is achieved.*

3. Place the phantom on the bucky, with the edge of the phantom aligned with the chest wall side of the image receptor. Position the phantom as if it were a breast. *Note: On the phantom there is a small indention to resemble the location of nipple, so make sure that this nipple marker is positioned away from the chest wall side of the image receptor.*

4. Lower the compression device down to bring the paddle in contact with the phantom.

5. Prepare to make the exposure, which should resemble the outcome of a 4–4.5 cm compressed breast. This may be done in two ways:

   a. If AEC is used, ensure that the phototimer detector is positioned under the phantom but is consistent in location with all previous phantom images.

   b. If the manual technique is used set the appropriate technical factors to be consistent with all previous phantom images.

6. Note and plot the exposure time on the chart after the exposure.

7. Process film.

8. Using the densitometer, measure the density on the film over the disk and then measure the background density adjacent to the disk. Be sure when measuring the background density that there are no fibrils interfering with the reading.

9. Plot the density of the background density on the control chart.

10. Plot the density difference (background density minus the density of the disk) on the control chart.

11. To score the phantom image, mask off any extraneous light from the image as if the radiologist were reading a mammogram. A magnifying lens may also be used for scoring.

12. Evaluate the film and determine how many simulated fibers, speck groups, and masses are visualized and record this on the control chart. To score the image:

    a. Count a mass as 1 point if it is identified within its correct location, its circular border is visible, and a density difference is noted.

    b. A mass is only awarded 0.5 point if it is identified within its correct location with a visible density difference but the circular border to the mass is not visible.

    c. Count the number of objects from the largest to the smallest.

    d. Each fiber is counted as 1 point if the entire fiber length is identified in the correct location.

    e. If only one-half of the fiber is visible but the fiber is identified in its correct location, it receives only 0.5 point.

    f. Speck groups consist of six individual specks. If four of the six specks are identified, the group is counted as 1 point.

    g. If only two or three specks are identifiable within a speck group, only 0.5 point is given to that speck group.

13. With the magnifying lens, evaluate the image for any areas that appear nonuniform and look for the presence of dirt or dust artifacts, grid lines, or any other artifacts to perform a comparative analysis with the original and previous phantom images. Indicate any of these artifacts by circling them on the film and subtracting one from the final total for each interfering artifact.

14. If artifacts are identifiable, investigate the artifact-causing source.

ANALYSIS

For a true analysis of the phantom images, it is important to maintain consistency. This evaluative test should always be performed and viewed by the same person with similar and consistent external factors concerned with the viewing and time of day the phantom is evaluated. For this test, it is important that one delegated person evaluates, scores, and charts the phantom images. However, other members within the department should also be asked to score the images on a routine if not a monthly basis. If a discrepancy in scores continues with the other evaluators from month to month or if there is a downward trend occurring in the scoring the QC technologist should determine the cause of this downward trend. This is when it is extremely helpful to rely on the original phantom and the previous phantom images to do an effective comparative analysis.

Several factors to evaluate for an acceptable outcome:

1. Film density should be greater than 1.2, with control limits of ± 0.20.

2. Density difference should be about 0.40, with control limits of ± 0.05 for a 4 mm thick disk.

3. Each phantom image must be scored and add up to a minimum of 10 points for the outcome to be within acceptable limits by ACR. ACR standards require that four fibers, three speck groups, and three masses be identifiable, equaling a minimum final total of 10.

4. For evaluation of the simulated test objects within the phantom, the results should not decrease by more than one-half assuming the same delegated QC technologist is performing and viewing the phantom images.

Other possible future problematic factors:

1. Any visual changes occurring between the current phantom image and the original film must be investigated.
2. If the density and the density difference readings exceed the suggested limits listed above, the processor, film batch, and generator should be investigated and corrective action taken.
3. If a continuous problem of visualization of grid lines, grid artifacts, artifacts, or the number of visualized simulated objects within the phantom is occurring, report this to the medical physicist for correction.

ACR requires that all phantom images be retained within the QC records for a full year.

Mammography Processor Quality Control

Processing plays an important role in film archival quality and for the production of film contrast and density. Through quality control, it is valuable to know that the dedicated processor for mammography films is functioning to the level of the manufacturer's specifications and that the processor's function is consistent. This daily quality control test requires the use of two separate pieces of equipment, a densitometer and a sensitometer. The densitometer is used to obtain readings of densities from specific areas on a film. Through plotting the required density readings, changes can be noted in contrast and speed. The sensitometer is used in the darkroom and exposes a scale of gray on a film, which gradually increases in density. The scale of gray exposed on a film is similar to the scale of gray created by a step wedge.

For accurate assessment of a processor's functioning, a quality control strip must be performed daily. For measurable outcomes, consistency plays a significant role. Quality control strips should be run each day before the arrival of patients or at least before any clinical mammograms are performed and processed. Evaluating the processor before it is in complete operation for the day allows for corrective action to be taken.

PURPOSE

To ensure that the processor is functioning to its specified maintainable limits and that the processor is consistent in its outcomes.

MATERIALS

Digital thermometer

Control box of mammographic film

Sensitometer (for mammography, the sensitometer should produce 21 steps in optical density in steps of 0.15)

Densitometer

Control chart

PROCEDURE

1. Check the temperature of the developer with a digital thermometer. Do not use a glass thermometer because the glass may break and the mercury may escape into the processor. The temperature must not differ by more than ±0.5°C from the manufacturer's specifications. Note the temperature on the control chart.

2. Take a piece of film from the designated control box and place the edge of the film into the sensitometer with the emulsion side down or as close as possible to the light source.

3. Process the film immediately with the emulsion side faced down and with the least exposed end of the strip fed through the processor first.

4. Be sure that the film is fed through the processor feed tray on the same side each day.

5. Using the densitometer, measure the following three areas and record on the control chart. Remember when measuring the steps on the sensitometric strip to always measure in the center of the step.

   a. Determine which sensitometric step has a density closest to 1.20. This step will be indicated as the medium density (MD), which is the speed indicator.

   b. Determine which sensitometric step has a density closest to 2.20.

   c. Determine which sensitometric step has a density closest to but not less than 0.45.

   d. Calculate the density difference (DD) by subtracting the result from step c or the density closest to but not less than 0.45 from step b or the density step closest to 2.20. Density difference is the contrast indicator.

   e. Take a density reading on any area of the film that has not been exposed by the sensitometer to obtain a base plus fog reading (B+F).

6. Record the MD, DD, and the B+F on the control chart.

If a QA program has not been established for the mammographic department, the delegated QC technologist must complete the initial start-up step. Before processor quality control begins, control numbers for the control chart must be achieved. This is accomplished by first designating a control box of film. Next, for the next 5 consecutive days, a sensitometric step must be run daily. From the daily sensitometric step, determine the MD, DD, and the B+F. After the 5 days are over, take the average of the MD, DD, and the B+F and chart these as the base control numbers.

ANALYSIS

If the plotted MD and DD fall within ±0.10 of the control limit and the B+F density is within ±0.03 of its control limit, the processor is functioning properly within its limits. However, if the MD and DD fall outside of the ±0.10 control limit but are contained within the ±0.15 limit, the test should be repeated immediately and the processor should be reevaluated for the possibility of human error. Furthermore, if the MD and DD fall outside of the ±0.15 control limit, the problem must be identified and corrected before the processor can be used for clinical use. As for B+F, if the outcomes exceed the ±0.03 control limit, corrective action must be taken immediately. On the control chart, any density readings that fall outside the control limits should be indicated by circling the plotted mark on the graph and by noting the possible cause of the problem in the designated area on the chart. When and if corrective action is taken, the test must be repeated and graphed to ensure that the result is within the control limits. Be observant of any day-to-day variations. If variations begin to show a trend, whether upward or downward, the source of the problem needs to be corrected.

Processor QC charts must be kept for a complete year, and the sensitometric films for the entire month prior must be retained.

Repeat Analysis

Reject analysis must be performed in every mammography department to track and identify any consistent problems that may occur from either positioning errors or equipment failure. Through this analysis, relevant factors can be improved, thereby improving department efficiency and reducing patient exposure. For a proper repeat analysis, all films that required an additional image and additional radiation dose to the patient must be included in the evaluation. A repeat analysis applies to all films, not just the films rejected by the radiologists.

A repeat analysis must start with any initial QC/QA program start-up. Thereafter, a repeat analysis data should be evaluated quarterly and recorded on the QC data sheet. To obtain a valid analysis, the mammography department should have a patient quantity of at least 250 during each quarter.

PURPOSE

To collect and evaluate data for the purpose of identifying any consistent problems that occur through mammographic positioning or equipment to determine the means for rejection.

MATERIALS

All rejected mammography films
QC data sheet

PROCEDURE

1. Gather the collection of films needed for evaluation for the quarterly period.
2. Calculate and determine the total number of film supply used during the quarterly period.
3. Calculate the total number of repeat films.
4. Calculate the total number of films exposed.
5. Sort the collection of films into categories by cause: (technique, positioning, artifacts, processing, good films that appear acceptable, etc.).
6. From each of these categories, calculate a total for each and record.

ANALYSIS

To calculate total number of repeat rates:

$$\text{Overall repeat rate} = \frac{\text{total number of rejected films}}{\text{total number of films exposed}}$$

To calculate the percentages of repeats in each category:

$$\% \text{ repeats/category} = \frac{\text{total repeats/category}}{\text{total repeats for all categories}}$$

Repeat rates based on a 250-patient volume indicate that the overall repeat rate should be less than 2%. Category repeats rates should not exceed 5%.

Screen Cleanliness

The quality of the mammogram is quickly degraded by the appearance of artifacts within the image. Artifacts such as dirt or dust have a tendency to mimic a microcalcification within the breast tissue. Through screen cleaning, mimicking artifacts can be reduced to a minimum, resulting in the avoidance of a repeat film to determine whether the calcification is in fact a calcification or dirt or dust artifact.

Screens should be cleaned weekly or when they are suspected of containing possible artifacts.

PURPOSE

To eliminate artifacts from a mammography screen that may mimic a possible pathology within the breast.

MATERIALS

Appropriate screen cleaning solution

Lint-free gauze pad or camel's hair brush

PROCEDURE

1. Remove films from screens and clean the insides of the screen. Be careful not to damage the screen by pressing too hard.
2. After cleaning the screen, set the cassette vertically and only slightly opened to allow the screen to dry before closing it.
3. Once the screen is dry, load the cassette with film and allow the cassette to set for at least 15 min to allow any trapped air to escape before use.

ANALYSIS

After cleaning the screen, evaluate its effectiveness through mammographic images. Technologists should determine whether a microcalcification is due to an artifact or pathology. Screens should be numbered individually to evaluate the microcalcification and its location on each film.

View–Box Uniformity

View boxes must be evaluated to ensure that viewing conditions are nothing less than optimum. One must maintain view boxes by evaluating the consistency across all view boxes within a mammography department. If the amount of illumination from the technologist's view box differs from that of the radiologist, image quality may not be optimum between the two viewing stations. This discrepancy affects the outcome of the mammographic diagnosis.

View boxes are evaluated by the amount of illumination and the optimum density and contrast ranges on films. Besides illumination, view boxes are evaluated for the overall cleanliness of the cover panel, light intensity, and the temperature of the color. The fronts of the view boxes must be cleaned of marks. The temperature of the color should be chosen to whatever hue is the most pleasing to the eye. All illuminators in each view box in each mammography department should be of the same brand and type to ensure consistent viewing conditions. All illuminators should all be replaced every 2 years. All fluorescent bulbs should be replaced at the same time to ensure uniformity. The intensity of the illuminators needs to be maintained. If an illuminator becomes dull, visibility of detail is reduced because of increased density appearance.

Contrast is important for the diagnosis of mammographic images. To improve contrast, extraneous light must be minimized so that it does not degrade the image quality. View boxes should be positioned in areas away from windows, sources of bright light, and other view boxes.

View box conditions should be analyzed weekly.

PURPOSE

To ensure that all viewing conditions are optimum and consistent to prevent a misdiagnosis.

MATERIALS

Window cleaner

Soft towel

PROCEDURE

1. Clean all view box surfaces until all marks are removed from the panel.
2. Visually inspect all view boxes for light uniformity.
3. Ascertain that any sources of extraneous light are not reflecting off of the view box fronts.

ANALYSIS

Evaluate the view boxes for uniformity and replace all bulbs at one time if dimming or flickering begins to occur within the bulbs. Ambient light and illuminator light can be measured with light meters. Ambient light refers to all the surrounding light conditions. Luminance is a measurement of the light intensity emitted from a view box. The illuminator light reading for mammography view boxes should register to at least 3500 nit, which will be higher than the luminance reading for diagnostic radiography. View boxes used for diagnostic radiography will have a luminance reading of 1500 nit.

Visual Checklist

Every month, mammography technologists should perform a visual checklist of the department's equipment. Technologists should be certain that all the buttons, peddles, displays, and lights are working properly, consistently, and are mechanically stable.

A visual checklist of the equipment must be performed monthly and after any equipment maintenance service on mammography units.

PURPOSE

To ensure that all aspects of the mammography unit is function properly to maintain the patient's safety and provide high-quality diagnostic films.

MATERIALS

Visual checklist according to the ACR manual

PROCEDURE

1. Grade the equipment by assigning a pass or fail check on the department's visual checklist after checking each function on the C-arm, cassette holder, and control booth.
2. For the C-arm portion of the checklist, check the SID indicator, the register of the C-arm angle, whether the locks work, whether the field light works, and whether the C-arm moves easily.
3. For the cassette holder portion of the checklist, check the cassette locks, grids, compression device, compression scale, and amount of compression delivered through manual and automatic modes.
4. For the control booth portion of the checklist, check the window, panel switches, lights, meters, and the technique charts.
5. Make sure that the mammography room is supplied with gonadal shielding, cones, and cleaning solutions.

ANALYSIS

Each item listed on the department's visual checklist must receive a passing grade. Items on the checklist that fail to meet the passing criteria need to be replaced immediately or serviced for correction.

CHAPTER 7

Artifact Assessment

ASSESSMENT

An artifact could be classified as any blemish visualized on a processed film. Artifacts can occur from processing, exposure, or handling/storage of film. Artifacts may occur on either single or double emulsion film; and in the instances in which the artifact interferes with the diagnostic quality of the film, the film must be repeated. Through repeat analysis, many departments catalog the number of reject films into categories to determine the nature of the repeats to eliminate or minimize the artifact from occurring before a trend begins to show-up. The formula for calculating repeat rate is as follows:

$$\text{Total repeat rate} = \frac{\text{number of repeated films} \times 100}{\text{total number of exposed films}}$$

Repeat rates should not exceed 4–6% for conventional radiography and should be less than 2% for mammography.

Artifacts can best be detected and eliminated if films are checked regularly. By identifying the possible causes for artifacts early, one can reduce the number of films that will be affected. Common sense tells us that this will provide us with the two benefits: reduced patient exposure and reduced operating costs.

To detect artifacts on a daily basis, one should always begin checking films before and after any processor preventative maintenance checks are performed or cleaning of any processor cross-over assemblies and before racks has occurred. One should also check for any artifacts on films as the film exits the processor. If an artifact is detected, try to isolate the cause for the artifact and make any corrections necessary to eliminate the artifact from occurring again.

The following sections include examples of common causes and appearance of processing, exposure, and handling/storage artifacts.

PROCESSING ARTIFACTS

DELAY STREAKS

Appearance   Wide, smooth bands without sharp edges. These bands may appear anywhere on the film parallel to the direction of film travel. The bands may have a plus density, minus density, or even a combination. The bands may occur on the first 3.14 in. of the film (one roller revolution) or may occur for two or three roller revolutions.

Cause   Bands may be due to a buildup of oxidized developer on the cross-over assembly due to improper processor ventilation.

Solution   Try running the designated roller clean-up film through the processor to control the delay streaks. Roller clean-up film will aid in removing lint, dirt, or other deposits. If you do not have access to specific clean-up film, use undeveloped fogged or expired film instead. To avoid contaminating the developer or redepositing dirt or lint, do not run the same film through the processor a second time. If this solution does not eliminate the delay marks, be sure to check that the developer tank is full, that the processor has adequate ventilation, and that the rollers are being adequately covered with solution.

ENTRANCE ROLLER MARKS

Appearance   Increased density bands are approximately 1/8-in. wide, which appear parallel to the direction of film travel. The entrance rollers cause marks as the film enters the developer.

Cause   Entrance roller marks may appear because of uneven pressure applied to the film as it passes through the rollers. Entrance roller marks may also result when there is an accumulation of moisture on the rollers because of inadequate processor ventilation or if films have already begun to feed through the rollers and then are pulled back out.

Solution   To eliminate entrance roller marks, open up the processor to ensure that the rollers are situated straight and are properly placed within their seats and check for adequate ventilation. Also, check to be sure that the entrance rollers are dry and clean.

GUIDE SHOE MARKS

Appearance   Guide shoe marks may occur as either increased or decreased density marks or scratches that run in the same direction or parallel to the film's direction of travel. Guide shoe marks occur at evenly spaced intervals and are commonly found at the leading and trailing edges of the film.

Cause   If there is evidence of increased density marks, it is most likely due to improperly seated guide shoes within the developer phase. If there is evidence of decreased density on the film but no signs of surface damage to the film, it is most likely due to improperly seated guide shoes in the fix-to-wash assembly rack. If there is evidence of decreased density and there are signs of surface damage to the film, this may denote a problem in the film transport path anywhere in the processor. Guide shoe marks also may appear if there is any chemical residue or deposit buildup on the guide shoes.

Solution   First, examine all the guide shoes in all the cross-over and turnaround assembly racks. Any guide shoes that appear worn, damaged, or bent should be replaced, and all rollers should appear straight. Also, check that all the guide shoe rollers are free from any built-up chemical debris.

CHATTER

Appearance   Increased density bands may differ in density, but they will be uniform in distance from one another. Chatter bands will appear perpendicularly to the film's direction of travel.

Cause   The transport component of the processor may not be functioning smoothly. The processor may be worn, out of alignment, damaged, or dirty.

Solution   Be sure the person in charge of maintaining the processor is completing the preventative maintenance checks. With regular maintenance, the processor should not suffer from much wear and tear.

DICHROIC STAIN

Appearance   The stain on a processed film has a brown and greenish-yellow color.

Cause   The appearance of the brown color indicates that either the developer is oxidized or hyporetention is present from years of storage. The greenish-yellow stain indicates the presence of undeveloped and unexposed silver halide crystals that were not properly removed from the film during processing.

Solution   Drain the developer and add fresh solution to the tank. Also, check the wash cycle to ensure that adequate washing of films is taking place to avoid hyporetention.

Brown Films

Appearance   Radiographs may appear to have a brown tint throughout or at random.

Cause   The first possibility for the production of brown stains or films is that the wash cycle may be functioning inadequately. The wash cycle may have an incorrect wash water level or inadequate water flow. The second possibility may be due to the fixer solution. The fixer solution could be depleted, of poor quality, improperly mixed, low in temperature, or the replenishment rate for the fixer solution may be set too low.

Solution   There are several. Make sure that the water filter does not need to be replaced, check the quality of the fixer solution, check the fixer replenishment rate, and check the temperature of both the water and the fixer solutions.

Emulsion Pick-off

Appearance   Small decreased-density spots on the film where the emulsion layer has been removed down to the base of the film.

Cause   Emulsion pick-off may result from poor processor upkeep. Rollers that become dirty and rough are responsible for removing the emulsion from the film. Pick-off may also be due to poor-quality or exhausted chemicals. Also, emulsion pick-off may be due to processing with underreplenished developer, causing glutaraldehyde failure.

Solution   Be sure to keep up with daily and monthly processor maintenance and supplying fresh chemicals to the tanks to maintain proper replenishment rates.

Skivings

Appearance   Thin threads of increased density marks represent emulsion that has been removed from and then redeposited on the film. Skivings may appear anywhere on the film but are usually seen about 3.14 in. from the leading edge of the film. Skivings may be detected visually on the surface of the film and by touch.

Cause   Skivings result when there is unsmooth transport of film, causing the rollers to remove a threadlike portion of emulsion from one area and then deposit the removed emulsion elsewhere.

Solution   Keep up with daily and monthly processor maintenance. Be sure that the appropriate chemical types and rates are being used for the selected film type (check the manufacturer's guidelines). Clean-up film may also be used to remove dirt and debris from the rollers.

Curtain Effect

Appearance   Solution runs or drips down the film as if the solution were a curtain. This effect is more common in films that are manually processed.

Cause   The curtain effect may occur in automatically processed films when a film jams in the processor and must be removed before drying. The curtain effect may also occur if the wash water is dirty.

Solution   Make sure that the transport system is functioning properly and that the wash water is clean.

Hyporetention

Appearance   Processed films may appear with a white powdery residue on the film's surface.

Cause   The film may have been insufficiently washed, resulting in the fixer solution not being completely removed from the film before drying.

Solution   Make sure that that the wash tank has adequate water levels; a clogged filter can cause insufficient water flow.

EXPOSURE ARTIFACTS

Exposure artifacts are caused by the patient, the technologist, or the equipment during a radiographic procedure. The following are examples of common artifacts that occur during the radiographic exposure.

MOTION

Motion on a radiograph is denoted by the blurry appearance. Motion may have been caused by an inadequately immobilized patient, the tube, or the image receptor.

ARTIFACTS

Artifacts may occur from either the patient or the ancillary equipment used for the procedure. Patient artifacts are classified as any radiopaque object that may be visualized from either inside or outside the patient's body. Ancillary equipment also contains artifacts. Artifacts could be inside cassettes or on positioning sponges (i.e., barium) and interfere with the production of the final image.

POOR FILM–SCREEN CONTACT

Poor film–screen contact may also cause localized blurring areas on a processed radiograph. Poor film–screen contact may result from dirty screens or old cassettes that are not making proper contact between the film and the screen.

GRID CUT–OFF

Grid cut–off appears as a decrease in optical density and is apparent when a grid absorbs a significant amount of the primary beam due to the misalignment between the tube and the grid. Misalignment may occur from using a grid improperly, e.g., inverted focused grid, improper tube angulation, lateral decentering, or an unleveled grid.

GRID LINES

Grid lines appear as areas of decreased density and are caused by absorption of the primary photons by the lead strips of the grid. Grid lines are most evident with low ratio grids, off-centering of the primary beam and grid, and stationary grids.

MOIRÉ EFFECT

The moiré effect resembles "double grid lines." Placing a grid within the bucky creates the moiré effect, which is usually most evident with low ratio stationary grids and the reciprocating bucky.

QUANTUM MOTTLE

Quantum mottle appears as variegated densities on the film. Quantum mottle is caused by differences in the photon energies reaching the image receptor and usually occurs at low settings.

STORAGE AND HANDLING ARTIFACTS

These types of artifacts occur during storage before use or from darkroom handling techniques.

AGE FOG

Age fog occurs when a film has been used for diagnostic exposure and processed after the film has expired. Age fog may also occur when the film is stored in an improper film environment. Any amount of age fog will cause the image to appear with lower contrast.

SAFELIGHT FOG

This type of fog results when safelights with improper bulb wattage are used, bulb filters are cracked, or when the safelights are placed at the improper distance from the work counter.

PRESSURE MARKS

Pressure marks appear most often in films that have been stored flat instead of vertically for a period of time. Because of the weight placed on the films before development, pressure marks occur and are identifiable as areas of increased optical density on a radiograph.

STATIC

Static may appear in three different patterns: tree, smudge, or crown. Each type of static pattern has its own characteristics. Static results when the humidity levels within the darkroom are inadequate. Low levels of humidity sparks patterns of electricity as films come into contact with other surfaces.

CRESCENT OR CRINKLE MARKS

These marks appear on processed radiographs as a direct result of improper film handling before development. These marks may appear as crescent moon shapes with increased density that result from bending of the film.

SHADOW IMAGES

Shadow images, commonly confused with emulsion pick-off, are small decreased density spots on a film that occur in a random pattern. Shadow images are most commonly noted on mammographic film, which is single emulsion. Shadow images are commonly caused by dirty cassettes and can be eliminated through regular screen cleaning maintenance. Also, working in a clean darkroom can minimize shadow images.

CHAPTER 8

Processor Quality Control

PROCESSOR QUALITY CONTROL

Automatic processors are complex systems that should be monitored regularly to ensure optimum performance. Processors should operate within tolerance levels allowed by the manufacturer. If any significant deviations from the specified tolerance levels occur, image quality will be affected. To maintain a processor's performance, regular preventative maintenance and scheduled cleanings should take place to minimize processor failure, artifact formation, and the production of poor-quality archived films. Processor manuals specify the daily, weekly, monthly, periodic cleaning, preventative maintenance procedures, and the appropriate start-up and shut-down procedures.

Items needed to perform daily processor quality control include:

- a clinical thermometer
- a simulated light sensitometer
- a control box of film
- a densitometer
- processor control charts

THERMOMETERS

Using appropriate thermometers is important when obtaining daily temperature read-outs. The clinical thermometer should have a reading range of 90–108°F and should not register any temperatures that fall below the lower specified limit of the thermometer. However, if the intention is to use the same thermometer to read developer, fixer, and wash solutions, a thermometer with a wider range should be obtained. Any thermometer that is made of glass should not be used because of the possibility of breakage.

When obtaining temperature readings for the purpose of daily monitoring, the thermometer, preferably digital, should be placed in the same location at the same time each day. Once the processor is heated to operating standards, a daily temperature reading should be obtained. Also, be sure that the probe of the thermometer is placed in the same spot each day because the recirculation system can cause a variation of as much as 1°F at different points within the developer tank. After each temperature check, the probe of the thermometer should be cleaned with warm water and dried to avoid processor contamination and to prolong the life of the thermometer.

SIMULATED-LIGHT SENSITOMETER

This device is used in the darkroom to expose an unprocessed film to different light intensities. The incremental difference between the light steps produced is usually set at about 0.15. Once the exposed film has been processed, it may be termed the *sensitometric strip,* the *processor QC strip,* or the *filmstrip.* The light emitted by the sensitometer will not be comparable to the light emitted by intensifying screens; thus, there will be a difference in the light recorded between the sensitometer and intensifying screens. With this in mind, simulated-light sensitometers should not be used to compare film speeds and contrasts with the film speeds and contrasts produced by intensifying screens.

Sensitometers produce a 21-step density strip specific to either single or double emulsion film. It is important to use the single-sided exposure setting for single emulsion films and a double-sided exposure setting for dual emulsion films. Also, when preparing the sensitometer for use, one should select the exposure made by the sensitometer to be sensitive to either blue or green film.

Sensitometers are used with the intention of producing a reproducible exposure, which in turn aids in daily processor monitoring. To meet this requirement of consistency, sensitometers should be stored in clean areas free from dust and dirt. To keep the exposure window of the instrument clean, canned air, which is free of moisture, may be used to keep this surface free of dust and dirt. *Note: Canned air should remain in the upright position during usage and should not be shaken prior to use.*

QUALITY CONTROL FILM

With the start-up of a processor quality control program, a fresh box of film should be selected and set aside for the purpose of processor monitoring only. The control box of film should be clearly labeled and stored in a place free of radiation, light, and chemical fog and in the appropriate temperature ranges. Mammography departments should have a dedicated processor specific for their mammography needs and should use that type of film for daily processor monitoring. For other processors that process a variety of film types, the most sensitive film should be used for daily sensitometric monitoring. No matter which type of film is used for daily processor monitoring, one film should be exposed by the sensitometer and run through the processor on the same side for 5 consecutive days, week after week. Once the control box of film is emptied, the QC technologist should perform a film cross-over with a new box of film.

To replace an existing control box of film and to eliminate variation from the process, the QC technologist must perform a cross-over technique from the old box of film to the new box of film. The QC technologist should perform the cross-over technique to make the appropriate changes to the operating levels on the control chart. The cross-over technique should be completed because film is produced in batches; thus, there will be slight variation in the outcomes of the sensitometric strips.

To perform a cross-over properly, the QC technologist should expose and process five films from both the old and the new boxes of film on the same day and at the same time of day, one film after another. From each film that is processed, values should be figured and averaged for B+F, the MD (reading closest to 1.20), the density reading closest to 2.20, and the density reading closest to but not less than 0.45 from the old and new boxes of film. After determining the averages of these values, the processor control chart may have to be adjusted to the new levels of B+F, the MD or speed index, and the DD or the contrast index that were figured.

Step 1 = average from new box of film − average from old box of film = difference

Step 2 = original operating level + difference = new operating level

When performing the cross-over technique, the processor should contain *seasoned chemicals* and not fresh chemicals. In other words, the chemicals should have been used previously to process film.

COMPONENTS OF PROCESSING

DEVELOPER

The developer is responsible for converting the latent image into the manifest image.

CHEMICAL MAKE-UP

The basic ingredients of the developer are solvents, developing or reducing agents, accelerators, preservatives, restrainers, and hardeners. To focus specifically on the reducing agents, there are the two standards ones: phenidone and hydroquinone.

Phenidone is the quick responsive agent that produces optical densities up to 1.2 on a film. Phenidone is the agent responsible for the minimum density (D_{min}) portion of the characteristic curve and the speed indicator. Hydroquinone is the slower responsive agent. Hydroquinone is responsible for completing the development process and creates optical densities greater than 1.2. Hydroquinone will also create the maximum density (D_{max}) portion of the characteristic curve and the contrast indicators needed for sensitometric testing. Hydroquinone is extremely sensitive to changes in temperature, concentration, and pH, and this agent is to first show signs of development failure. It is important to remember that the measurable optical densities on a film are due to the action of synergism or *superaddivity.* Synergism is the action of these chemicals working together more efficiently than alone.

TEMPERATURE CONTROL

The temperature of the developer may have a range of 90–100°F, depending on the manufacturer's specifications. Developer solutions can deviate by ±0.5°F from the set standard. Temperature monitoring should be completed daily with sensitometric monitoring to ensure that the processor is functioning properly on a day-to-day basis. Temperature monitoring should be completed at the same time and in the same place everyday with an appropriate clinical digital thermometer.

Note: Developer temperatures that remain lower than the specified target temperature will result in the reduction of the film's speed, resulting in additional and unnecessary radiation doses given to the patient to produce radiographs with similar optical densities. Conversely, if the temperatures are above the specified target temperature, the speed of the film is increased, resulting in lower radiation doses and increased film contrast.

FIXER

The fixer removes the remaining unexposed and undeveloped silver halide crystals from the film, completes the development stage, and hardens the film for storage purposes.

CHEMICAL MAKE-UP

The fixer solution is composed of the fixing (hypo or thiosulfate), preservative, hardener, buffer, and sequestering agents. The fixation cycle of development must clear the undeveloped silver ions from the film to ensure proper long-term storage. Incomplete fixation may not become evident until the image has been stored for a certain period. Hyporetention tests for radiography should be obtained every 6 months and quarterly for mammography through the use of a commercial hyporetention kit. The ANSI recommends that the acceptable limit of residual hypo be less than 2 μg/cm^2 for diagnostic radiography and 5 μg/cm^2 for mammography.

TEMPERATURE CONTROL

The temperature of the fixer may be 85–95°F and can deviate from the manufacturer's set standards by ±5°F. The temperature of the fixer is not as crucial as that of the developer. A higher temperature reading for the fixer solution results in improved fixation and generally does not cause any problems.

WASH CYCLE

The wash cycle should remove any remaining traces of chemicals from the film and prepare the film for long-term storage. Sufficiently removing remaining chemicals from the film will prevent fading and any film discoloration over time.

TEMPERATURE CONTROL

Water stabilizes the temperatures of the other processing solutions. Some processors use cold and hot water or *water-controlled systems,* in which the temperature is regulated by a mixing valve. Other processors may operate with cold water entering the processor which then must be routed through a heating element. This type of system is referred to as a *thermostatically controlled system.* The control of wash water temperature is not as crucial as the developer or fixer temperature. However, there are control limits that must be applied to units that use cold water and heating elements. In many processors, the units that operate with cold water use the cold water to cool the developer. In these instances, the cold water should be heated to 5–10°F below the temperature of the developer. As for the temperature of the incoming cold water, it should be lower than 40°F. Water temperatures should be maintained at 40–85°F.

DRYING

The final phase of processing the film is the drying phase. The dryer section of the processor uses heated air. Most of the air supplied to the processor will be recirculated; the rest may be vented out to prevent a buildup of excessive humidity within the dryer section.

TEMPERATURE CONTROL

Dryer temperature should be set as low as possible but should ensure adequate drying of the films. Dryer temperatures should be set to and not exceed the requirements set by the film manufacturer's recommendations. Typically, heat ranges of 1500–3000 W power and the dryer is set to control temperatures of 100–160°F.

pH Measurement

The pH measurement determines the concentration of hydrogen ions in the solution. Using pH measurements for chemical solutions is not very accurate for detecting small insufficiencies in the chemical's function but may be useful for detecting trends or great changes. An incorrect pH reading indicates an improperly mixed solution, but a correct pH reading is not the final indicator for properly mixed solutions. Solution concentration is as follows:

pH for developer solutions = 10–11.5
pH for fixer solutions = 4–4.5

Solution pH should not differ from the manufacturer's specifications by more than ±0.1.

Specific Gravity

Specific gravity is a unitless value obtained by the ratio of comparing the density of the *x* liquid with the density of water. Specific gravity measurements are obtained for the purpose of ensuring that proper dilution of solutions has been made but not for each individual component within the solution. Specific gravity measurements can be obtained through the use of a hydrometer. For accurate readings of specific gravity with the hydrometer, be sure to obtain the measurement of specific gravity at the temperature to which the hydrometer was calibrated. Specific gravity measurements are as follows:

Developer solutions:	range of 1.07–1.1 and should not differ by more than ±0.004
Fixer solutions:	range of 1.077–1.11 and should not differ by more than ±0.004

Charting Processor QC

Processing plays an important role in film archival quality and in the production of film contrast and density. With quality control, the dedicated processor for mammography films will function at the manufacturer's specifications and will function consistently. This daily quality control test requires the use of two separate pieces of equipment: a densitometer and a sensitometer. The densitometer is used to obtain readings of densities from specific areas on a film. Through plotting the required density readings, changes can be noted in contrast and speed. The sensitometer is used in the darkroom and exposes a scale of gray on a film, which gradually increases in density. The scale of gray exposed on a film is similar to the scale of gray created by a step wedge.

Consistency plays a significant role, for accurate assessment of the processors functioning. A quality control strip must be produced and evaluated daily. Quality control strips should be run each day before the arrival of patients or before any clinical radiographs are performed and processed. Evaluating the processor before it is in complete operation for the day allows for corrective action.

PURPOSE

To ensure that the processor is functioning to its specified maintainable limits and that the processor is consistent in its outcomes.

MATERIALS

Digital thermometer

Control box of radiographic film

Sensitometer

Densitometer

Control chart

PROCEDURE

1. Check the developer temperature with a digital thermometer. Do not use a glass thermometer due to possible glass breakage causing mercury to contaminate the processor. The temperature must not differ by more than $\pm 0.5°C$ from the manufacturer's specifications. Note the temperature on the control chart.

2. Take a piece of film from the designated control box and place the edge of the film into the sensitometer with the emulsion side placed next to the light source.

3. Process the film immediately with the emulsion side face down and with the least exposed end of the strip fed through the processor first.

4. Be sure that the film is fed through the processor feed tray on the same side each day.

5. With the densitometer, measure the following three areas and record on the control chart. When measuring the steps on the sensitometric strip, always measure in the center of the step.

    a. Determine which sensitometric step has a density closest to 1.20. This step is the MD, or speed indicator.

    b. Determine which sensitometric step has a density closest to 2.20.

    c. Determine which sensitometric step has a density closest to but not less than 0.45.

    d. Calculate the DD by subtracting the result from step c or the density closest to but not less than 0.45 from step b or the density step closest to 2.20. DD is the contrast indicator.

    e. Take a density reading on any area of the film that has not been exposed by the sensitometer to obtain a B+F reading.

6. Record the MD, DD, and the B+F on the control chart.

If a QA program has not been established for the radiology department, the delegated QC technnologist must complete the initial step. Before processor quality control begins, control numbers for the control chart must be obtained, which is accomplished by first designating a control box of film. Next, for the next 5 consecutive days, a sensitometric step must be run daily. From the daily sensitometric step, figure the MD, DD, and the B+F. After the 5 days are complete, take the average of the MD, DD, and the B+F and chart these as the base control numbers.

ANALYSIS

If the plotted MD and DD fall within ±0.15 of their control limits and the B+F density is within ±0.03 of its control limit, the processor is functioning properly within its limits. However, if the MD and DD fall outside of the ±0.15 control limit, the test should be repeated immediately and the processor should be reevaluated with regard to human error. Furthermore, if MD and DD fall outside of the ±0.15 control limit, the problem must be identified and corrected before the processor can be used for clinical use. As for B+F, if the outcomes exceed the ±0.03 control limit, corrective action must be taken immediately. On the control chart, any density readings that fall outside the control limits should be indicated by circling the plotted mark on the graph and noting the possible cause of the problem in the designated area on the chart. When and if corrective action is taken, the test must be repeated and graphed to ensure that the result is within the control limits. Watch for day-to-day variations. If variations begin to show a trend, whether upward or downward, the source of the problem needs to be corrected.

Processor QC charts must be kept for a complete year, and the sensitometric films for the entire month prior must be retained.

The sensitometric curve is also referred to as the *characteristic curve,* the *H & D curve,* and the *D-log E curve.* It is a graphical representation of the response the film has to specific exposure factors and processing conditions.

It is important to understand the five basic components of the curve. Components include B+F, the toe portion, the straight-line portion, the shoulder portion, and the D_{max}. Each component is influenced by something specific and contributes to a particular portion of the curve and thus the image.

BASE AND FOG

The B+F is consists of inherent film densities. Inherent film densities include those that are put into the film during the manufacturing process such as dyes, tints, and any intrinsic fog. The inherent density of B+F for unprocessed film is 0.05–0.1 and that for processed film is 0.1–0.25. The B+F may also be referred to as the $D_{min,}$ or minimum density.

TOE

The toe portion of the curve is the region just above the threshold. Recorded densities for this region usually range between 0.25 and 0.50. The reducing agent phenidone controls the toe. This part of the curve is sensitive to low density or little exposure, which may include bone, scatter, lead markers, and areas of high photon absorption.

STRAIGHT-LINE PORTION

The most useful densities, or those that contribute most to the image, are recorded as the straight-line portion of the characteristic curve. The straight-line portion is located between the toe and the shoulder. It includes densities between 0.5 and 2.5, but those that provide the most information are recorded in the 0.5–1.25 range. The straight-line portion is graphed in a linear fashion and indicates the speed. There is a direct relation between the densities recorded and the length of exposure.

SHOULDER

Hydroquinone is the reducing agent that contributes to the shoulder portion of the curve. This is the portion of the curve where the number of recorded densities cease. The shoulder is usually encountered at 2.5–3.0.

D_{MAX}

D_{max} is the top portion of the shoulder, or the point at which the maximum density is recorded. After D_{max}, solarization occurs. Silver halides are fully balanced once this maximum density is achieved and no more silver atoms can be accepted.

INTERPRETING THE CHARACTERISTIC CURVE

GAMMA

Gamma a characteristic of the straight-line portion of the curve. It is represented by a lateral drift or moving of the straight line to the right. The more vertical the straight-line portion of the curve, the less gamma recorded or fewer shades of gray. This is interpreted as a higher scale of contrast. The more horizontal drift recorded in the straight-line portion, the more shades of gray or gamma, which is interpreted as a longer scale of contrast.

SPEED

The speed of the curve is the amount or number of densities recorded during a given exposure. The more sensitive a film is to exposure, the greater the number of useful densities it will record. The faster the film reacts to a given exposure, the more sensitive it is. Films that react more quickly to an exposure will record a greater number of densities than slower films at the same exposure. Film speed or sensitivity is defined as the exposure required to produce a given density.

AVERAGE GRADIENT

The average gradient is defined as the slope of the straight-line portion of the curve and is a graphical representation of the contrast of the image. The average gradient exists within the straight-line portion of the characteristic curve. We can graph the average gradient by drawing a straight line from D_{min} to the point at which the useful densities of the straight-line portion stop (usually at 2.25). We then find the slope or degree of these two angles. This represents the average gradient. The steeper or greater the average gradient, the higher the contrast of the image. The less the average gradient, the lower the scale of contrast.

LATITUDE

Latitude is the range of exposure factors, which will produce densities that create a diagnostic image. Because a greater range of exposures usually produces an image with less contrast, the relation between contrast and latitude is inverse. As latitude, or the range of allowable exposures, increases, the contrast of the image decreases. The opposite is also true. High contrast images are usually produced within a limited range of exposures or with little latitude.

SILVER RECOVERY

The Resource Conservation and Recovery Act (RCRA) was passed to protect the health of humans and the environment. One requirement many facilities are required to perform is the collection of the unexposed silver from film from the processor chemicals. Not only does this benefit the environment; it also provides the facility with an additional source of revenue. There are a number of techniques available for silver recovery from processing solutions, but the three most practical methods are electrolysis, metallic replacement, and precipitation.

- Through the process of *electrolysis,* a direct current is passed through a silver-rich solution. Once the current has submerged into the fixer, an electron is transferred from the cathode to the positively charged silver, causing the silver to convert to its metallic state and stick to the cathode. Electrolysis recovers silver in its almost pure metallic state. One advantage of this method is that it allows for the reuse of the fixer solution according to the manufacturer's standards for the processor.

- The *metallic replacement method* is the simplest and the least expensive route to silver recovery. However, the reuse of solutions is not an option with this method. With this method, a steel-wool cartridge is placed within a canister. The iron within the steel wool reacts with the acid and silver ions within the fixer solution, causing an ion exchange to occur. From the chemical reaction of the acid in the fixer solution and the iron, metallic silver is formed.

- The *precipitation method* of silver recovery is the oldest form of recovery and is not as widely used as the other two methods. This method allows the silver to settle to the bottom of the solution, where it then can be removed. This method involves more direct contact with the hazardous chemicals and fumes and undoubtedly it is labor intensive.

MATERIAL SAFETY DATA SHEET (MSDS)

HAZARDOUS CONTROL OF CHEMICALS

The Occupational Safety and Health Administration (OSHA) has put forth several regulations to address health and safety issues within medical facilities across the United States. One OSHA regulation has made employees aware of chemical hazards present within their facilities. OSHA developed regulations based on the principle facts that (a) all employees are entitled to be made aware of any hazards that are present within the facility and (b) all employees are entitled to the right of protection from any chemical hazards present within the facility. This specific regulation covers issues such as hazard evaluation, MSDSs, chemical lists, chemical/container labels, and training for those employees who use are in direct contact with the chemicals.

The purpose of OSHA's Hazard Communication Standard is to educate and communicate any of the possible chemical hazards to which an employee may be exposed. Besides informing the facility's own employees, the facility is also responsible for communicating hazardous situations with outside individuals who come into the facility to perform a job or function. These individuals may be vendors or maintenance workers. In addition to the OSHA Hazard Communication Standard, some states have a "Worker's Right-to-Know" law that entitles employees to additional education on chemical hazards.

One component of the Hazard Communication Program that medical facilities are required to have is the MSDS. MSDSs are to be developed for each chemical manufactured or imported by the manufacturer. MSDS material should be available in the appropriate language and must contain the following information for each chemical:

- Identification of the hazardous components in the chemical
- The chemical and physical characteristics
- Any possible health effects from exposure
- The limits of exposure to the chemical
- The primary routes of chemical entry
- Precautionary and control measures for the chemical
- Prepared identification
- Preparation date of the chemical
- Emergency treatment information

MSDSs must be kept on file for each chemical and must be readily accessible to all employees. *A rating scale of severity consists of four levels: level 4 is considered the most severe, whereas level 1 is considered a slight hazard.*

CHAPTER 9
Statistical Analysis

METHODS OF ANALYZING DATA

Statistical Basics

POPULATION

Identifying the population to be measured is the first step in TQM. The population is defined as the group or set that is being measured. Conditions specific to the population are usually evaluated singularly.

SAMPLE

A sample is a portion of a population that represents the population. Sampling allows for data to be collected about the population by measuring a given number of the population. This is also known as *choosing a portion, variable,* or *evaluating a subset* of the general population. It is a much more efficient way to evaluate large populations such as radiology outpatients. When sampling, one must evaluate how much and when to obtain the sample to reduce variability and ensure accuracy.

CONTINUOUS VARIABLES

Continuous variables have no end. They have limitless ranges of mathematical values. An example of a continuous variable is height.

DICHOTOMOUS VARIABLES

A dichotomous variable allows for two choices. An example of a dichotomous variable is beef or chicken.

DATA SET

The information or measurements acquired by evaluating the sample is termed the *data set*. Because the entire population has not been evaluated, we infer the results of the sample on the entire population. This is termed *data* or *statistical inference.*

Mathematical Description

FREQUENCY

The frequency of an event is calculated by counting the specific number of observations of the event within a category.

CENTRAL TENDENCY

The central tendency is the midpoint of the frequency of a sample. The three things that can be used to measure the central tendency are the mode, mean, and median.

MODE

The mode is the measurement that occurs most repeatedly.

MAXIMUM

The maximum is the largest value detected.

MINIMUM

The minimum is the smallest value detected.

MEAN

The mean is commonly referred to as the average value. The mean is calculated by finding the sum of all the detected values and dividing that number by the total number of detected values.

MEDIAN

The median is the numerical middle. It has an equal number of values that is greater than and less than itself.

STANDARD DEVIATION

The standard deviation (or SD) is defined as the range of variation around the mean and is often signified by the letter sigma (σ). According to Poisson statistics, one may obtain the standard deviation by finding the square root of the mean.

$$SD = \sqrt{\frac{\sum x^2}{N}}$$

When large variations occur, the following possibilities should be considered:

- This may be a normal occurrence.
- The system being evaluated is not within limits.
- The way the measurements were obtained, calculated, or determined may be incorrect.

VARIANCE

Variance is the square root of the standard deviation. Variance is applied when comparing the standard deviation of several groups.

TOOLS FOR PROBLEM IDENTIFICATION AND ANALYSIS

The use of statistical tools is an integral part of the application of TQM in any type of manufacturing or service industry. These tools are helpful in the design, implementation, and maintenance phases of TQM. Statistical tools allow for data to be collected on processes, which then can be charted and further analyzed for improvement purposes.

There are seven basic statistical tools, each serving a specific purpose, that can be used for the interpretation and analysis of data:

Flowcharts

Run charts

Control charts

Histograms

Pareto diagram

Cause-and-effect diagram

Scatter diagram

Flowcharts

To understand the problems inherent in a process, one must first understand how the complete process works. By understanding how a process works, one can identify any problem areas that create variation within the system. Eliminating the identifiable inconsistencies can always reduce variations. Flowcharts are best developed when people who are actually involved within the process construct the flowchart. These people may include employees, managers, supervisors, and customers. Once the flowchart is complete, team members are able to identify any quality problems and areas in need of improvement.

There are specific standards and symbols that characterize a flowchart. When constructing a flowchart, one must identify all the inputs, outputs, and actions and chart these items in the order in which they occur. Remember to construct a detailed chart of the entire process from start to finish in basic steps. When constructing the flowchart, one must also characterize each step with the appropriate symbol. The symbols are represented as follows:

A rectangle represents the activity symbol. Only include a brief description of the activity.

A diamond represents decision, i.e., the point at which a decision is made within a process. This point may divide the process into two or more paths.

An oval or rectangle is used to denote the terminating point within a process or the starting point of a process.

A flow line is a symbol that represents the path or connection between the steps of a process. The arrowhead on the flow line indicates the direction of the process.

Run Charts and Control Charts

Control of processes is a continuous activity and requires that measurements be taken periodically during the process. With run and control charts, one can visually display the process, any variation within the process, and, most importantly, determine the point where a process goes out of control.

Run charts, also referred to as *trend charts,* map data in a linear fashion over a period of time. The vertical axis represents the measurement, and the horizontal axis denotes the time scale. Run charts display the performance and any variation of a process over a given period. Run charts can be used to graphically display production volumes or costs, for example. Run charts also provide the user with a visual display of any changes or variation within a process over time and display the effects of any corrective action taken toward variation within the process.

The first step in constructing a run chart is to identify the measurement or indicator that is to be monitored. Next, the collection of relevant data must be obtained. Once data collection is complete, one should examine the range of data collected. Scale the chart so all the data can be plotted on the vertical axis. Be sure to leave some additional room for any new data that may be collected later on. The third step involves plotting all the data on the chart and connecting the

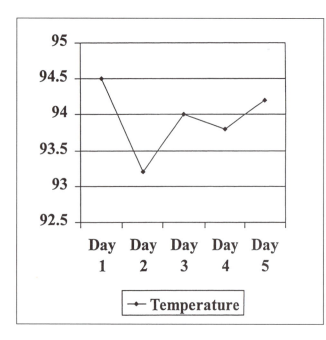

FIGURE 9-1

plotted points with a linear line. Finally, determine the average of all the plotted points and create the center line, which runs horizontally, on the chart through the average of plotted points.

After completing the chart, evaluate the plotted points. If the points fluctuate in a stable pattern around the center line, without any large spikes or trends (upward or downward movements), the process is under control. If unusual patterns are noted within the plotted points, an investigation for the lack of stability should be performed.

Control charts are simple run charts with two horizontal lines, or control limits, added to the chart. The control chart consists of an upper control limit and a lower control limit. The control chart, similar to a run chart, displays the performance of any process desired over time. From the graphical display, one can determine whether the process is consistent and operating within its statistical limits.

If plotted sample data fall outside of the control limit or if nonrandom patterns exist within the chart, then the process is unstable. The entire process should be reevaluated and corrective action taken. Control charts are unable to determine the source of any problem within a process. Alternative problem-solving mechanisms should be applied to determine the root cause of the problem.

Histograms

A histogram is a simple bar graph. Histograms graphically represent the random variation in a given set of data. The height of each bar on the vertical axis represents the frequency or the number of observations made for the subject under analysis.

Histograms can fall into several typical patterns. Its symmetrical shape resembles a bell. The process is centered on a specified central value, which tapers off to be less frequent as one moves away from the

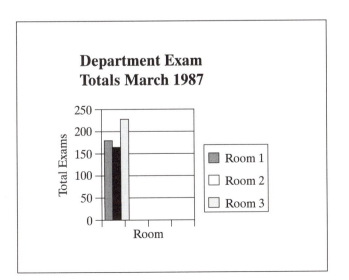

Department Exam Totals March 1987

FIGURE 9-2

central value. A *bimodal* pattern occurs when two groups of bell-shaped measurements are combined. The bimodal pattern represents a wide variability within the data, but there is no central tendency. A *skewed* pattern is similar to the bell-shaped pattern, but it is not symmetrical. The distribution of data tends to trail off in one direction.

Pareto Diagrams

A Pareto diagram, named after Wilfredo Pareto, is a histogram of the data graphically charted from the largest to the smallest frequency. The largest frequency is placed on the left side of the chart, which then decreases to the smallest frequency, on the right. A Pareto chart may be helpful in selecting a project for improvement based on priority. Pareto diagrams also aid in representing the results of improvement programs/techniques applied over a given period.

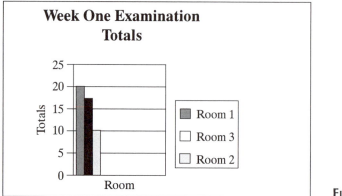

FIGURE 9-3

Cause-and-Effect Diagrams

This tool is effective for identifying the causes of problems, generating ideas for problem causes, and finding solutions for the problem. Because of the graphical appearance of this diagram, it is commonly referred to as the *fishbone diagram.*

An individual or, preferably, a team can construct cause-and-effect diagrams. Through team application, brainstorming becomes the facilitator. Teams enable the participants to focus on the issue and immediately brainstorm for the causes of the final effect.

When constructing a cause-and-effect diagram, one first must determine the quality characteristic to be improved. Second, team members can brainstorm to generate ideas as to what is causing the effect. These ideas become the main causes and are listed on branches flowing toward the main branch of the diagram. Third, the team must continue to brainstorm on all the possible problems for each major cause category for the entire diagram. These ideas are listed as subcauses within each cause branch.

Scatter Diagrams

Scatter diagrams, unlike the previous tools listed, represent the relations between paired data that are acquired when analyzing a process. The previous statistical tools are capable of handling only one type of data at a time. With scatter diagrams, one is able to plot corresponding groups of collected data and plot them respectively. Typically, scatter diagrams can be correlated from cause-and-effect diagrams.

Once the data variables are plotted on the x and y axes, one should examine the plot to determine whether the correlation between the points is positive or negative. If the correlation is positive, there will be an increase in variable x in relation to an increase in variable y. If the correlation is negative, there will be an increase in variable x in relation to a decrease in variable y. If the plotted points do not represent any type of linear relation, then there is no correlation between points.

DECISION-MAKING TOOLS FOR GROUPS

Teamwork is one element in the success of any TQM program. Individuals rarely have enough knowledge or experience to completely understand all the aspects of the most important organizational processes. Thus, team approaches tend to be the most effective for process improvements. A *team* consists of at least two people; the ideal number in any team is 6–12. Teams are concerned with a particular task for which all the team members are equally accountable. The most effective teams are those who are goal-centered, independent, open, and empowered by management. Through teamwork, individuals within the organization are empowered to develop new processes or improve old processes and continually monitor their improvement efforts. There are many types of teams and methods in different organizations to identify problems, to collect and analyze data, to improve processes, and to improve customer satisfaction. The following types of teams and methods are discussed:

Focus groups

Quality improvement teams

Quality circles

Problem-solving teams

Work teams

Brainstorming

Consensus

Multivoting

Focus Groups

Focus groups are small groups that focus on finding a solution to any particular problem. This panel of individuals may take approaches such as brainstorming, interviewing customers or noncustomers, or taking surveys to understand a problem within a process that may affect customer satisfaction. Through surveys and customer comment cards, focus groups can provide the true voice of the customer. However, focus groups may have higher implementation costs compared with other approaches.

Quality Improvement Teams

The purpose of a quality improvement team is to implement the solutions the focus groups have determined will improve a particular process.

Quality Circles

Quality circles are usually composed of workers and supervisors who come from the same department or have the same function. This small group of people meets regularly to identify, solve, and implement solutions to organizational problems. Quality circles may also be in place to discuss departmental problems concerning issues such as departmental quality and levels of productivity.

Problem-Solving Teams

A problem-solving team is an example of a cross-functional team in which team members meet to solve particular problems. Cross-functional teams are those that work on specific tasks and in doing so cut across the horizontal rather than vertical boundaries of other departments to complete tasks. Problem-solving teams identify, analyze, and solve quality and productivity issues. Team members are taught the appropriate problem-solving tools by team leaders and are guided by a facilitator.

Work Teams

Work teams focus on completing an entire task or solving a complete problem rather than focus on a particular step in a process. When these teams are fully empowered by management, they are referred to as *self-managed teams* (SMTs). SMTs are composed of 6–18 well-trained professionals and are responsible for completing specifically defined quality of work. SMTs are empowered and are responsible for taking corrective action on any issues that directly concern their purpose as a team. SMTs are able to resolve their own day-to-day problems, access any information needed to implement a plan, and control or improve the focus of their operations. SMTs have become the most popular and advanced concept in teamwork. Organizations have found that, through the use of SMTs, both the employee and the organization benefit. SMTs facilitates continuous improvement, creates greater employee involvement and job satisfaction, increases organizational commitment and morale, and aids in the recruitment and retention of the best people.

Brainstorming

Brainstorming is a method used in group settings to generate ideas and possible solutions for the decision-making process. The facilitator of a brainstorming session should encourage participation and discussion relevant to the matter at hand and keep a record of all the ideas generated. To conduct a successful brainstorming session, the facilitator should:

- Announce the topic to be discussed to all team members before the session
- Begin the session by reviewing the subject at hand
- Phrase the topic to be discussed in the form of a question
- Allow the group to work together to generate ideas or divide the group into smaller groups to promote idea generation
- Be sure that all ideas are recorded
- Encourage the expansion of ideas from the best suggestions

Consensus

After a brainstorming session, an idea list should be compiled and, through consensus, a final idea should be decided. Through consensus, a team must work toward an agreement on the best action to take from the entire list of suggestions. Consensus does not require total agreement, but the decision should at least be acceptable to each member. However, in reaching consensus, each member should be allowed to voice concerns on the matter. This may in fact stimulate discussion arising from opposing opinions or identifiable conflicts.

Multivoting

The multivoting method may be used to dismiss unessential ideas and concentrate on the essential ones. This method is accomplished by listing all the issues that were brainstormed and allow all the members to vote on which issues are the most important. Next, all the votes should be tallied, and the ideas with the fewest votes should be discarded. This method should be repeated until only a few ideas remain for discussion. Once the list has been shortened, the remaining ideas should be voted upon to determine the one idea for discussion.

DATA COLLECTION METHODS AND INDICATORS

Since the United States quality revolution in the 1980s, many organizations have learned to focus on the customer in response to the competitive market. It is crucial in today's market for competitive success that organizations fully understand what consumers want and need. Customer satisfaction occurs when services or products at least meet or go beyond the customer's expectations. Customer dissatisfaction results from poor-quality products or services and leads to customer complaints, returns, loss of business, and jeopardizes the retention of other customers due to the publicity made by unsatisfied customers. Customer retention is a complementary factor of customer satisfaction.

The goal of any of any organization should be to meet and exceed the customer's needs and expectations. A customer can be defined as any person or department who wishes to obtain a desired outcome. Customers can be defined more specifically as internal customers and external customers. Internal customers, when referring to the health care industry, may be any of the following: employees of a health care organization, whether they are individual or departmental employees; departments; and referring physicians. Generally speaking, internal customers are staff and coworkers within the facilities. External customers may be any of the following: patients, families of patients, or third-party payers.

The voice of the customer is an essential way to making quality improvement efforts. However, capturing the thoughts and delineating the appropriate changes can be challenging because the customers' needs and wants are continually changing. However, there are some key approaches that may be useful in gathering customer information.

Customer Cards and/or Surveys　This approach may be the simplest way to obtain customer information. However, for this approach to be effective, the questionnaire should produce valid and reliable information that will also generate a high response rate. When formulating a questionnaire, be sure that:

1. It is brief and to the point
2. The questionnaire can be completed within 15 min
3. The same questionnaire is administered to each individual
4. Questions must be measurable quantitatively (multiple choice or Likert scale)
5. Surveys should always be pretested to determine whether or not the instructions are understandable

Written surveys tend to be the most common means of measuring satisfaction levels, but other techniques such as telephone interviews and face-to-face interviews may be used through focus groups. Written surveys generally involve a lower data collection cost and easier analysis. However, written surveys are disadvantageous because of a high nonresponse bias and they require a larger volume of surveys to be administered.

Focus Groups   Focus groups may be composed of a panel of individuals who may be either customers or noncustomers. These panels of individuals work to answer questions about the organization's service or products and questions about competitor services or products. Focus groups may use interview techniques to capture the true voice of the customer through direct interaction.

Focus groups that use either face-to-face or phone interview techniques are advantageous because they allow for a much smaller sample size to generate qualitative information. However, these techniques have higher costs and increased time commitments.

With the results of either approach, complaints or comments can be analyzed to learn about product or service failures. Even though the complaints are undesirable data, organizations can form cross-functional teams to collect more data and analyze the problems that are occurring, especially between the organization's goals/expectations and the actual performance interaction with the customers. Through team organization, employees may be empowered with the responsibility for developing appropriate improvement plans in response to customer complaints. Once new processes have been implemented to improve the unsatisfactory areas, organizations should follow up with another survey and analyze the new results. These new processes should be surveyed every 3 months until the improved process has proved to be stable. By using this technique, we are actually incorporating customer feedback into the CQI concept.

To satisfy customers, organizations should:

- Focus on and understand the customer's needs and wants
- Increase overall organizational rather than departmental performance
- Analyze processes within the organizations and work to reduce any unnecessary variation that decreases levels of quality produced
- Empower teams to seek new and improved ways to meet and exceed customer expectations
- Educate organizational employees continually
- Use problem-solving techniques to detect and reduce sources of variation within the organization's system

TQM/CQI organizations should work to provide internal and external customer satisfaction. Providing satisfaction will rely heavily on the commitment of the entire organization working toward a common goal. Quality management principles focus on satisfying the internal customers first for the delivery of products or services to the external customer at the highest quality level. Further, customer satisfaction measurements should not be restricted to the external customers. Information gained from internal customers will also aid in a true assessment of the organization's overall strengths and weaknesses.

In the industry of health care, perception plays a large role in gaining customer satisfaction and retention. Perceptions and customer expectations represent the voice of the customer within the community. There are three levels of quality on which industries should focus to deliver quality products and services: perceived, expected, and actual. *Perceived quality* is based on the customer's perception of the product or service. The customer's perceptions are highly subjective to the type of advertisement regarding the product or service. *Expected quality* is based on the actual customer's experience with the product or service and level of satisfaction. *Actual quality* is not as easily measured as perceived or actual quality because it is based more on facts and numbers. These facts and numbers represent the comparison of product or service quality with that of a competitor.

In health care, there are some specific set standards that act as performance indicators for measuring levels of quality:

- *Appropriateness of care* represents the determinant of whether a certain type of care is necessary.
- *Continuity of care* represents how well the course of care administered is coordinated.
- *Availability of care* refers to how available a certain type of care or treatment is for a patient at a clinical facility.
- *Safety in the care environment* represents the factor of safety throughout the facility, whether it is competency in the staffs' abilities, application of universal precautions, or equipment operation.
- *Effectiveness of care* refers to the benefits obtained from the service under ordinary circumstances from the average worker.
- *Efficacy of care* refers to the benefits gained through the offering of health care services under the ideal conditions and above-average circumstances.
- *Efficiency of care* refers to the outcome obtained when high health care standards are administered in a short period and that benefit the organization and the customer with decreased expense and positive results for the patient.

CHAPTER 10

Federal Regulations

NATIONAL COUNCIL ON RADIATION PROTECTION AND MEASUREMENTS

Report Number 99: Quality Assurance for Diagnostic Imaging Equipment

This report specified why quality assurance programs should be established in health care facilities, what quality assurance programs can secure for the consumer and the worker, and what the suggested content of a quality assurance program should include.

The most important aspects of this report to the quality management personnel are those that deal directly with increasing quality and consistency of images within the imaging department. Quality assurance programs specify levels of performance for personnel. It is a management tool that gathers and evaluates data particular to human performance and function. Although these data may also involve equipment application by personnel, the evaluation of equipment is primarily considered to be part of a quality control program.

Four factors have been suggested by the National Council on Radiation and Protection (NCRP) for improving departmental performance and assuring high-quality personnel performance:

- Identifying those conditions within the department that require personnel to make decisions or take an action.
- Enact policies that guide personnel in the actions to be taken.
- Encourage adherence to the policy through recognition and education.
- Study in detail and at regular intervals the department's operation records.

Other important aspects of NCRP Report Number 99 include sections 6 and 7, which specify the required parameters for quality control of all processing and equipment maintenance. This report applies to the imaging physician and physicist and to the technologist.

Report Number 105: Radiation Protection for Medical and Allied Health Personnel

This report specifically concerns personnel who work directly with radiation or sources of radiation. Information contained within the report addresses the needs and requirements of the worker in addition to basic information about radiation.

The most important aspects of this report to radiology personnel are those that deal directly with defining exposure units and quantities, exposure limits for workers and patients, sources of radiation, and principles of protection from radiation.

Radiology technologists and the requirements for this occupation are found in section 8.4 of the document. As a quality management specialist, it is important to have a firm understanding of the regulations and definitions. The NCRP has noted the need for supervisors to be aware of possible hazards the worker may encounter when using radiation within the clinical environment. The NCRP also defines some very important terms such as *ALARA, should, shall,* and possible sources of exposure within the clinical environment.

The sections of most concern to the quality management specialist are 1, 2, 5, 6, and 7, in addition to section 8.4.

Appendices

APPENDIX 1
Quick Reference to Test Frequency for Radiography

Test	Frequency
Tube filtration	Annually
Reproducibility	Annually
Radiation output	Annually
Timer accuracy	Annually
Focal spot	Annually
Kilovoltage	Annually
Voltage waveform	Annually
Wire mesh	Annually
Portables/mobile equipment	Annually
Screen condition	Semiannually
Beam restriction	Semiannually
Field light congruence	Semiannually
PBL	Semiannually
Fixer retention	Semiannually
ANSI/wash	Semiannually or quarterly
Safelight	Semiannually
View box	Change bulbs every 2 years
Film duplicator	Inspect weekly

ANSI, American National Standards Institute.

APPENDIX 2

Quick Reference to Test Frequency for Mammography

Test	Frequency
Darkroom cleanliness	Daily
Screen cleaning	Weekly
View boxes	Weekly
Viewing conditions	Weekly
Phantom	Monthly
Visual inspection	Monthly
SID	
Angulation indicator	
Field light	
Compression	
Repeat analysis	Quarterly
Archival quality/hypo	Quarterly
Darkroom fog	Semiannually
Film–screen contact	Semiannually
Compression	Semiannually
Physicist survey	Annually
FDA inspection	Annually
Collimation	Annually
Skin entrance dose	Annually
Beam quality	Annually
Phantom image scoring	Annually

FDA, Food and Drug Administration;
SID, source-to-image distance.

NOTES

NOTES

NOTES

NOTES

NOTES

NOTES

NOTES

NOTES

NOTES

NOTES

Competency Documentation
Radiographic Critique and Interpretation

Date completed	Facility name	Patient identification	Verifying official

*A minimum of 50 documentations is required and must be completed under the supervision of the interpreting radiologist.

Competency Documentation
Radiographic Critique and Interpretation

Date completed	Facility name	Patient identification	Verifying official

*A minimum of 50 documentations is required and must be completed under the supervision of the interpreting radiologist.

Competency Documentation
Mammography Examinations

Date completed	Facility name	Patient identification	Verifying official

*A minimum of 100 documentations is required.

Competency Documentation
Mammography Examinations

Date completed	Facility name	Patient identification	Verifying official

*A minimum of 100 documentations is required.

Competency Documentation
Mammography Examinations

Date completed	Facility name	Patient identification	Verifying official

*A minimum of 100 documentations is required.

Competency Documentation
Mammography Examinations

Date completed	Facility name	Patient identification	Verifying official

*A minimum of 100 documentations is required.

Competency Documentation
Special Mammographic Procedures

Date completed	Facility name	Observe/participate	Verifying official

*A minimum of two special procedures is required. One can either participate or observe any of the following: needle localization, ductography, fine-needle aspiration, MRI, ultrasound, or stereotactic biopsy.

Competency Documentation
Compression Test

Date completed	Facility name	Equipment/room	Verifying official

*A minimum of one compression test is required.

Competency Documentation
Darkroom Cleanliness

Date completed	Facility name	Equipment/room	Verifying official

*A minimum of 25 documentations is required.

Competency Documentation
Darkroom Fog

Date completed	Facility name	Equipment/room	Verifying official

*A minimum of one documentation is required.

Competency Documentation
Film–Screen Contact

Date completed	Facility name	Equipment/room	Verifying official

*A minimum of one documentation is required.

Competency Documentation
Fixer Retention Test

Date completed	Facility name	Equipment/room	Verifying official

*A minimum of one documentation is required.

Competency Documentation
Phantom Imaging

Date completed	Facility name	Equipment/room	Verifying official

*A minimum of four documentations is required.

Competency Documentation
Processor Quality Control

Date completed	Facility name	Equipment/room	Verifying official

*A minimum of 20 documentations is required.

Competency Documentation
Repeat Analysis

Date completed	Facility name	Equipment/room	Verifying official

*A minimum of one documentation is required.

Competency Documentation
Screen Cleanliness

Date completed	Facility name	Equipment/room	Verifying official

*A minimum of four documentations is required.

Competency Documentation
View Box Uniformity

Date completed	Facility name	Equipment/room	Verifying official

*A minimum of three documentations is required.

Competency Documentation
Visual Checklist

Date completed	Facility name	Equipment/room	Verifying official

*A minimum of one documentation is required.

Automatic Exposure Control and Density Control Functions

Date completed	Facility name	Equipment/room	Verifying official

*Two competencies are required.

Timer Accuracy and Reproducibility

Date completed	Facility name	Equipment/room	Verifying official

*Two competencies are required.

Half Value Layer

Date completed	Facility name	Equipment/room	Verifying official

*Two competencies are required.

Grid Uniformity of Exposures

Date completed	Facility name	Equipment/room	Verifying official

*Two competencies are required.

Light Field Congruency

Date completed	Facility name	Equipment/room	Verifying official

*Two competencies are required.

MA Linearity

Date completed	Facility name	Equipment/room	Verifying official

*Two competencies are required.

Output Reproducibility

Date completed	Facility name	Equipment/room	Verifying official

*Two competencies are required.

Kilovoltage Reproducibility

Date completed	Facility name	Equipment/room	Verifying official

*Two competencies are required.

Screen–Film Contact

Date completed	Facility name	Equipment/room	Verifying official

*Two competencies are required for 24 cassettes tested.

Darkroom Fog

Date completed	Facility name	Equipment/room	Verifying official

*Four competencies are required.

Fixer Retention

Date completed	Facility name	Equipment/room	Verifying official

*Four competencies are required.

Phantom Image Evaluation

Date completed	Facility name	Equipment/room	Verifying official

*Four competencies are required.

Image Artifact Cause Evaluation

Date completed	Facility name	Equipment/room	Verifying official

*Four competencies are required.

Darkroom Cleanliness

Date completed	Facility name	Equipment/room	Verifying official

*Ten competencies are required.

Processor Quality Control Charting

Date completed	Facility name	Equipment/room	Verifying official

*Two months of charting and interpretation are required.

H & D Curves

Date completed	Facility name	Equipment/room	Verifying official

*Produce and interpret sensitometric curves for at least two different film types.

Problem Solving

Date completed	Facility name	Equipment/room	Verifying official

*Two competencies are required, involving any of the following: quality improvement teams, focus groups, brainstorming, flowcharts, cause-and-effect diagrams, histograms, Pareto charts, trend charts, or control charts.

Evaluate Shielding Devices

Date completed	Facility name	Equipment/room	Verifying official

*Two competencies are required. Fluoroscopy may be done on lead gloves, aprons, thyroid shields, goggles, or any type of gonadal shield.

Develop Radiographic Technique Charts

Date completed	Facility name	Equipment/room	Verifying official

*One chart is required.

View Box Evaluation

Date completed	Facility name	Equipment/room	Verifying official

*Evaluation should be done on one bank of view boxes for cleanliness, luminance, consistency of luminance, and illuminance.

Data Collection

Date completed	Facility name	Equipment/room	Verifying official

*Collect data on two indicators by using at least two of the following: questionnaire, patient records, focus groups, logs, or diaries.

Analyze and Display Data

Date completed	Facility name	Equipment/room	Verifying official

*Analyze and display data collected by using each of the following tools: flowcharts, cause-and-effect diagrams, scatter plots, histograms, Pareto charts, trend charts, control charts, and run charts.

Data Analysis Methods

Date completed	Facility name	Equipment/room	Verifying official

*Conduct analysis, interpret results, formulate analysis reports summarizing data from at least one indicator: counts, percentages, ratios, rates, mean, median, mode, range, standard deviation, and variance.